Bedtime Journal

For a good night's sleep and a better tomorrow

The power of bedtime journalling

Achieving a good night's sleep is an art. We spend approximately a third of our lives asleep so that the mind, body and soul can deeply rest, recharge and be replenished. When we do what we can to get a good night's sleep it doesn't only affect how we sleep, but also how we feel the next day.

Creating a period of time between the day and night; when you can put the pressures of the day behind you and prepare yourself for a good night's sleep, is one of the most powerful ways of experiencing all its benefits and maintaining your balance and wellbeing. This time and space can help you to process your day and the experiences you had and put aside any worries, fears or difficult thoughts that may otherwise seek your attention during your sleeping hours, so that it's easier to switch off and get a good night's sleep.

The physical benefits of getting enough sleep are well known, but sleep powerfully benefits our emotional and mental health too. After a good night's sleep we feel calmer and can think more clearly and make better decisions. When we're well rested we are less reactive and can handle more pressures. We feel better able to cope and life is less stressful as a result. It's also easier to stay present after a good night's sleep so we're more likely to have more energy and give to ourselves and others in the way we want to.

This bedtime journal will help you prepare for a good night's sleep by supporting you to consciously create a distinction between your day and sleep time. Repeating these exercises for the next 90 days can help them to become a natural part of your bedtime routine supporting a positive attitude and aligning you more closely with the life you want to lead.

The following pages will help you understand the importance of these practices and there is an example on the first page to give you an idea of what you can include, remember this is your journal and your responses will be unique to you.

Preparing for sleep is one of the most powerful ways to take care of your emotional health and wellbeing, supporting you to get a better night's sleep and wake up feeling refreshed and energised, ready for a new day.

Reflecting on your day

When we give ourselves the chance to reflect on experiences we've had and how they affected us as they happen, it allows us to learn what we need from them and move on. If you've not had the chance to pause throughout the day, you might find that your mind becomes very active at night when you try and sleep, as it tries to do this when you've finally stopped and have no other distractions around you. If your mind takes a long time to slow down and switch off, writing your thoughts down before you go to bed can help it to quieten down.

Each day you will have the space to think about what went well. It's often easy to overlook the positive parts of your day, what you did that you're happy with or proud of and focus on the opposite, but having a negatively biased perspective can lead to stress, worry and low mood. Taking the time to think about what went well in your day, what you enjoyed and what was beneficial to you can help you to become more comfortable recognising your strengths and the positives in your day and thus help you maintain a balanced perspective.

We all have strengths and weaknesses or limitations and if we only focus on our strengths and ignore our current limitations then this can create problems too. Each day, there is space for you to think about what didn't go well during your day, when you reacted in ways you'd rather not, so you can think about what you'd like to do differently in the future. Learning from difficult experiences by focusing on what you want to improve, rather than ruminating on what you did in the past or beating yourself up about it, is far more helpful. This perspective can help you grow and develop a more supportive and compassionate relationship with yourself, so you feel calmer and more relaxed and more able to get a good night's sleep.

Tuning in to your emotions

This journal can help you to become more attuned to your feelings and how they are influencing you; your thoughts, decisions and actions. Becoming comfortable and accomplished at tuning into yourself and your emotions will help you to better understand and support yourself.

We are using the terms 'emotions' and 'feelings' interchangeably to refer to the way you feel; your internal reaction. Your emotions may be loud and impossible to ignore, stopping you from living life the way you want to or they might sit quietly underneath the surface, not getting in your way but a constant nagging feeling making it hard to feel truly happy.

Our emotions are signals, they are designed to help us interpret the world around us and respond accordingly so that we can stay safe and thrive. Sometimes the emotions we experience are based on our physical reality, but more often than not they are are based on our thoughts about it rather than the situation itself. Regrets about the past, worries about the future, disappointments, a fear of failure, lack or being rejected can all create difficult emotions in us that can hold us back. Tuning in to your emotions at the end of each day will give you the space to process and move on from them, helping you to get a good night's sleep and wake up feeling more relaxed the next day.

When we name and write down our emotions it can give us some distance from them. Here are some examples of common feelings you may have:

Angry	Anxious	Jealous	Disappointed	Happy
Irritated	Scared	Disgusted	Empty	Loving
Annoyed	Fearful	Guilty	Sad	Amazed
Frustrated	Frightened	Embarrassed	Concerned	Glad
Furious	Stressed	Humiliated	Overwhelmed	Excited
Relaxed	Calm	Ashamed	Numb	Proud

Practising gratitude

Practicing gratitude, meaning consciously focusing on the things that you have in your life that you're thankful for, has been found to have profound effects on the mind and body.

Many situations that we find ourselves in will have both positive parts, that suit us well as well as other parts that we're not so happy about or that we could do without.

When we focus on the parts that are difficult or what we don't have but really want, it's easy to feel sad and unsupported. Over time, these feelings can spiral robbing us of motivation and creating feelings of depression and hopelessness. When, instead, we focus on the parts that are going well and what we do have whether that's our health, friends, family, a safe home or being able to feed our family, then we feel more hope, joy and happiness despite the challenges we might be facing.

Practising gratitude helps us feel calmer and happier with our lot. Even better, it's been shown that when practised over time it shapes what we focus on and the way that we naturally think, so that life becomes easier and more satisfying. An attitude of gratitude doesn't just affect the way we feel though, it also affects our physical body and has been shown to reduce inflammation and improve sleep (amongst other benefits).

Each day, you have the space to think about 5 things that you are grateful for a practice which is designed to help you develop a natural tendency to focus on the positives in your life. Taking the time to really recognise how you feel about these things, or what life would be like without them, can help you to feel genuinely grateful for them.

Setting intentions

Energy flows where attention goes and this is at the heart of intention setting. When we set intentions we're thinking about how we'd like our life to be, fine-tuning our desires and influencing the direction of our future.

Science shows us that our brains change and adapt according to our experiences and as the power of the mind is so strong, it doesn't matter if these experiences are real or imagined. When we spend time imagining the experiences that we want, our brains will slowly attune to them, making them more likely to happen. This same process happens if we focus on the experiences that we don't want, which is why intention setting is so important.

The mind and body are intrinsically linked and directing the thoughts we have by setting intentions has been shown to influence the biochemical processes that occur in the body. If we set positive intentions about our sleep, our cells will act in accordance with this, making it more likely we will fulfil them. When we set intentions about how we want to feel the following day, the same is also likely.

Intentions need to be truly felt and believed to create this effect on the body. If it's hard to believe the intentions you are setting will happen, instead try and imagine how this will feel in your body if it does.

Each day you will have the space to think about your bedtime intentions e.g. to sleep deeply or to remember your dreams. Over time, with continued practice setting and believing in the reality of your intentions, this will shape the connections formed in your brain, making it more likely these will become your new reality.

Equally, by thinking in advance about what we want to do differently tomorrow, we are more likely to make that our reality too.

Preparing for a good night's sleep

Many factors influence how well we sleep. Make sure to leave enough time before bed to properly prepare yourself for a good night's sleep:

Avoid big meals before going to sleep. Large and heavy meals e.g. those that include meat or other hard to digest foods require a lot of energy to process. If you eat these shortly before going to bed your body will invest its energy in digesting them instead of replenishing and rebalancing your body.

Avoid screens before bed. TVs, smart phones and other screens emit blue light which suppresses the secretion of melatonin making it harder to transition into sleep and get good quality rest. The body can also secrete high levels of Dopamine in response to what you're watching which can make it harder to drift off and get uninterrupted sleep.

Create an environment conducive to sleep. A calm environment will help your mind and body relax and at the end of the day. Making sure that your room is dark and relatively cool and removing all electronic equipment can also help.

Shower before bed. This helps to cleanse and wash away the day. The bodies cooling response, after a warm shower, can help you to drift off more easily.

Practise breathing exercises. Breathing exercises help the body to recognise that it's safe helping you relax. The more relaxed you feel, the easier it is to drift off to sleep more quickly.

Bedtime journal. Reflecting on and letting go of the pressures from your day and setting intentions for how you want your sleep and the following day to be, sends your mind, energy and focus in the direction you want it to go, allowing you to benefit fully from a good night's sleep.

What went well today?

1. Had a lovely phone chat with Sara
2. Supported myself to stay calm in a difficult meeting
3. Became playful, not angry, with the kids at dinner

5 things I'm grateful for..

1. Having two beautiful and healthy children in my life
2. A supportive partner who's there for me when I need
3. Food in the fridge
4. A warm house for me and my family
5. Seeing my family at the weekend

Intentions for my sleep tonight..

1. To sleep deeply so my body can best replenish and heal
2. To remember my dreams and understand their messages
3. To wake up in the morning with the energy I need

What do I want to do differently tomorrow?

1. Take regular breaks at work, not on my phone
2. Stay calm getting the kids out on time
3. To get into bed before 10pm

Date __ / __ / 20__

What went well today?

1. _____
2. _____
3. _____

5 things I'm grateful for..

1. _____
2. _____
3. _____
4. _____
5. _____

Intentions for my sleep tonight..

1. _____
2. _____
3. _____

What do I want to do differently tomorrow?

1. _____
2. _____
3. _____

Date __ / __ / 20__

What went well today?

1. _____
2. _____
3. _____

5 things I'm grateful for..

1. _____
2. _____
3. _____
4. _____
5. _____

Intentions for my sleep tonight..

1. _____
2. _____
3. _____

What do I want to do differently tomorrow?

1. _____
2. _____
3. _____

What went well today?

1. _____
2. _____
3. _____

5 things I'm grateful for..

1. _____
2. _____
3. _____
4. _____
5. _____

Intentions for my sleep tonight..

1. _____
2. _____
3. _____

What do I want to do differently tomorrow?

1. _____
2. _____
3. _____

Date __ / __ / 20__

What went well today?

1. _____
2. _____
3. _____

5 things I'm grateful for..

1. _____
2. _____
3. _____
4. _____
5. _____

Intentions for my sleep tonight..

1. _____
2. _____
3. _____

What do I want to do differently tomorrow?

1. _____
2. _____
3. _____

What went well today?

1. _____
2. _____
3. _____

5 things I'm grateful for..

1. _____
2. _____
3. _____
4. _____
5. _____

Intentions for my sleep tonight..

1. _____
2. _____
3. _____

What do I want to do differently tomorrow?

1. _____
2. _____
3. _____

Date __ / __ / 20__

What went well today?

1. _____
2. _____
3. _____

5 things I'm grateful for..

1. _____
2. _____
3. _____
4. _____
5. _____

Intentions for my sleep tonight..

1. _____
2. _____
3. _____

What do I want to do differently tomorrow?

1. _____
2. _____
3. _____

What went well today?

1. _____
2. _____
3. _____

5 things I'm grateful for..

1. _____
2. _____
3. _____
4. _____
5. _____

Intentions for my sleep tonight..

1. _____
2. _____
3. _____

What do I want to do differently tomorrow?

1. _____
2. _____
3. _____

What went well today?

1. _____

2. _____

3. _____

5 things I'm grateful for..

1. _____

2. _____

3. _____

4. _____

5. _____

Intentions for my sleep tonight..

1. _____

2. _____

3. _____

What do I want to do differently tomorrow?

1. _____

2. _____

3. _____

Date __ / __ / 20__

What went well today?

1. _____
2. _____
3. _____

5 things I'm grateful for..

1. _____
2. _____
3. _____
4. _____
5. _____

Intentions for my sleep tonight..

1. _____
2. _____
3. _____

What do I want to do differently tomorrow?

1. _____
2. _____
3. _____

Date __ / __ / 20__

What went well today?

1. _____
2. _____
3. _____

5 things I'm grateful for..

1. _____
2. _____
3. _____
4. _____
5. _____

Intentions for my sleep tonight..

1. _____
2. _____
3. _____

What do I want to do differently tomorrow?

1. _____
2. _____
3. _____

Date __ / __ / 20__

What went well today?

1. _____
2. _____
3. _____

5 things I'm grateful for..

1. _____
2. _____
3. _____
4. _____
5. _____

Intentions for my sleep tonight..

1. _____
2. _____
3. _____

What do I want to do differently tomorrow?

1. _____
2. _____
3. _____

Date __ / __ / 20 __

What went well today?

1. _____
2. _____
3. _____

5 things I'm grateful for..

1. _____
2. _____
3. _____
4. _____
5. _____

Intentions for my sleep tonight..

1. _____
2. _____
3. _____

What do I want to do differently tomorrow?

1. _____
2. _____
3. _____

Date __ / __ / 20__

What went well today?

1. _____
2. _____
3. _____

5 things I'm grateful for..

1. _____
2. _____
3. _____
4. _____
5. _____

Intentions for my sleep tonight..

1. _____
2. _____
3. _____

What do I want to do differently tomorrow?

1. _____
2. _____
3. _____

Date __ / __ / 20__

What went well today?

1. _____
2. _____
3. _____

5 things I'm grateful for..

1. _____
2. _____
3. _____
4. _____
5. _____

Intentions for my sleep tonight..

1. _____
2. _____
3. _____

What do I want to do differently tomorrow?

1. _____
2. _____
3. _____

Date __ / __ / 20__
_____

What went well today?

1. _____
2. _____
3. _____

5 things I'm grateful for..

1. _____
2. _____
3. _____
4. _____
5. _____

Intentions for my sleep tonight..

1. _____
2. _____
3. _____

What do I want to do differently tomorrow?

1. _____
2. _____
3. _____

Date __ / __ / 20__

What went well today?

1. _____
2. _____
3. _____

5 things I'm grateful for..

1. _____
2. _____
3. _____
4. _____
5. _____

Intentions for my sleep tonight..

1. _____
2. _____
3. _____

What do I want to do differently tomorrow?

1. _____
2. _____
3. _____

Date __ / __ / 20__

What went well today?

1. _____
2. _____
3. _____

5 things I'm grateful for..

1. _____
2. _____
3. _____
4. _____
5. _____

Intentions for my sleep tonight..

1. _____
2. _____
3. _____

What do I want to do differently tomorrow?

1. _____
2. _____
3. _____

Date __ / __ / 20__

What went well today?

1. _____
2. _____
3. _____

5 things I'm grateful for..

1. _____
2. _____
3. _____
4. _____
5. _____

Intentions for my sleep tonight..

1. _____
2. _____
3. _____

What do I want to do differently tomorrow?

1. _____
2. _____
3. _____

What went well today?

1. _____
2. _____
3. _____

5 things I'm grateful for..

1. _____
2. _____
3. _____
4. _____
5. _____

Intentions for my sleep tonight..

1. _____
2. _____
3. _____

What do I want to do differently tomorrow?

1. _____
2. _____
3. _____

Date __ / __ / 20__

What went well today?

1. _____
2. _____
3. _____

5 things I'm grateful for..

1. _____
2. _____
3. _____
4. _____
5. _____

Intentions for my sleep tonight..

1. _____
2. _____
3. _____

What do I want to do differently tomorrow?

1. _____
2. _____
3. _____

Date __ / __ / 20__

What went well today?

1. _____
2. _____
3. _____

5 things I'm grateful for..

1. _____
2. _____
3. _____
4. _____
5. _____

Intentions for my sleep tonight..

1. _____
2. _____
3. _____

What do I want to do differently tomorrow?

1. _____
2. _____
3. _____

What went well today?

1. _____
2. _____
3. _____

5 things I'm grateful for..

1. _____
2. _____
3. _____
4. _____
5. _____

Intentions for my sleep tonight..

1. _____
2. _____
3. _____

What do I want to do differently tomorrow?

1. _____
2. _____
3. _____

Date __ / __ / 20__

What went well today?

1. _____
2. _____
3. _____

5 things I'm grateful for..

1. _____
2. _____
3. _____
4. _____
5. _____

Intentions for my sleep tonight..

1. _____
2. _____
3. _____

What do I want to do differently tomorrow?

1. _____
2. _____
3. _____

Date __ / __ / 20__

What went well today?

1. _____
2. _____
3. _____

5 things I'm grateful for..

1. _____
2. _____
3. _____
4. _____
5. _____

Intentions for my sleep tonight..

1. _____
2. _____
3. _____

What do I want to do differently tomorrow?

1. _____
2. _____
3. _____

Date __ / __ / 20__
_____

What went well today?

1. _____
2. _____
3. _____

5 things I'm grateful for..

1. _____
2. _____
3. _____
4. _____
5. _____

Intentions for my sleep tonight..

1. _____
2. _____
3. _____

What do I want to do differently tomorrow?

1. _____
2. _____
3. _____

What went well today?

1. _____
2. _____
3. _____

5 things I'm grateful for..

1. _____
2. _____
3. _____
4. _____
5. _____

Intentions for my sleep tonight..

1. _____
2. _____
3. _____

What do I want to do differently tomorrow?

1. _____
2. _____
3. _____

Date __ / __ / 20__

What went well today?

1. _____
2. _____
3. _____

5 things I'm grateful for..

1. _____
2. _____
3. _____
4. _____
5. _____

Intentions for my sleep tonight..

1. _____
2. _____
3. _____

What do I want to do differently tomorrow?

1. _____
2. _____
3. _____

Date __ / __ / 20__

What went well today?

1. _____
2. _____
3. _____

5 things I'm grateful for..

1. _____
2. _____
3. _____
4. _____
5. _____

Intentions for my sleep tonight..

1. _____
2. _____
3. _____

What do I want to do differently tomorrow?

1. _____
2. _____
3. _____

What went well today?

1. _____

2. _____

3. _____

5 things I'm grateful for..

1. _____

2. _____

3. _____

4. _____

5. _____

Intentions for my sleep tonight..

1. _____

2. _____

3. _____

What do I want to do differently tomorrow?

1. _____

2. _____

3. _____

Date __ / __ / 20__

What went well today?

1. _____
2. _____
3. _____

5 things I'm grateful for..

1. _____
2. _____
3. _____
4. _____
5. _____

Intentions for my sleep tonight..

1. _____
2. _____
3. _____

What do I want to do differently tomorrow?

1. _____
2. _____
3. _____

Date __ / __ / 20__

What went well today?

1. _____
2. _____
3. _____

5 things I'm grateful for..

1. _____
2. _____
3. _____
4. _____
5. _____

Intentions for my sleep tonight..

1. _____
2. _____
3. _____

What do I want to do differently tomorrow?

1. _____
2. _____
3. _____

Date __ / __ / 20__
_____

What went well today?

1. _____
2. _____
3. _____

5 things I'm grateful for..

1. _____
2. _____
3. _____
4. _____
5. _____

Intentions for my sleep tonight..

1. _____
2. _____
3. _____

What do I want to do differently tomorrow?

1. _____
2. _____
3. _____

What went well today?

1. _____
2. _____
3. _____

5 things I'm grateful for..

1. _____
2. _____
3. _____
4. _____
5. _____

Intentions for my sleep tonight..

1. _____
2. _____
3. _____

What do I want to do differently tomorrow?

1. _____
2. _____
3. _____

Date __ / __ / 20__

What went well today?

1. _____
2. _____
3. _____

5 things I'm grateful for..

1. _____
2. _____
3. _____
4. _____
5. _____

Intentions for my sleep tonight..

1. _____
2. _____
3. _____

What do I want to do differently tomorrow?

1. _____
2. _____
3. _____

Date __ / __ / 20__

What went well today?

1. _____
2. _____
3. _____

5 things I'm grateful for..

1. _____
2. _____
3. _____
4. _____
5. _____

Intentions for my sleep tonight..

1. _____
2. _____
3. _____

What do I want to do differently tomorrow?

1. _____
2. _____
3. _____

Date __ / __ / 20__

What went well today?

1. _____
2. _____
3. _____

5 things I'm grateful for..

1. _____
2. _____
3. _____
4. _____
5. _____

Intentions for my sleep tonight..

1. _____
2. _____
3. _____

What do I want to do differently tomorrow?

1. _____
2. _____
3. _____

Date __ / __ / 20__
_____

What went well today?

1. _____
2. _____
3. _____

5 things I'm grateful for..

1. _____
2. _____
3. _____
4. _____
5. _____

Intentions for my sleep tonight..

1. _____
2. _____
3. _____

What do I want to do differently tomorrow?

1. _____
2. _____
3. _____

What went well today?

1. _____
2. _____
3. _____

5 things I'm grateful for..

1. _____
2. _____
3. _____
4. _____
5. _____

Intentions for my sleep tonight..

1. _____
2. _____
3. _____

What do I want to do differently tomorrow?

1. _____
2. _____
3. _____

Date __ / __ / 20__

What went well today?

1. _____

2. _____

3. _____

5 things I'm grateful for..

1. _____

2. _____

3. _____

4. _____

5. _____

Intentions for my sleep tonight..

1. _____

2. _____

3. _____

What do I want to do differently tomorrow?

1. _____

2. _____

3. _____

Date __ / __ / 20__

What went well today?

1. _____
2. _____
3. _____

5 things I'm grateful for..

1. _____
2. _____
3. _____
4. _____
5. _____

Intentions for my sleep tonight..

1. _____
2. _____
3. _____

What do I want to do differently tomorrow?

1. _____
2. _____
3. _____

What went well today?

1. _____

2. _____

3. _____

5 things I'm grateful for..

1. _____

2. _____

3. _____

4. _____

5. _____

Intentions for my sleep tonight..

1. _____

2. _____

3. _____

What do I want to do differently tomorrow?

1. _____

2. _____

3. _____

Date __ / __ / 20__

What went well today?

1. _____
2. _____
3. _____

5 things I'm grateful for..

1. _____
2. _____
3. _____
4. _____
5. _____

Intentions for my sleep tonight..

1. _____
2. _____
3. _____

What do I want to do differently tomorrow?

1. _____
2. _____
3. _____

Date __ / __ / 20__

What went well today?

1. _____
2. _____
3. _____

5 things I'm grateful for..

1. _____
2. _____
3. _____
4. _____
5. _____

Intentions for my sleep tonight..

1. _____
2. _____
3. _____

What do I want to do differently tomorrow?

1. _____
2. _____
3. _____

Date __ / __ / 20__

What went well today?

1. _____
2. _____
3. _____

5 things I'm grateful for..

1. _____
2. _____
3. _____
4. _____
5. _____

Intentions for my sleep tonight..

1. _____
2. _____
3. _____

What do I want to do differently tomorrow?

1. _____
2. _____
3. _____

Date __ / __ / 20__

What went well today?

1. _____
2. _____
3. _____

5 things I'm grateful for..

1. _____
2. _____
3. _____
4. _____
5. _____

Intentions for my sleep tonight..

1. _____
2. _____
3. _____

What do I want to do differently tomorrow?

1. _____
2. _____
3. _____

Date __ / __ / 20 __

What went well today?

1. _____
2. _____
3. _____

5 things I'm grateful for..

1. _____
2. _____
3. _____
4. _____
5. _____

Intentions for my sleep tonight..

1. _____
2. _____
3. _____

What do I want to do differently tomorrow?

1. _____
2. _____
3. _____

Date __ / __ / 20__

What went well today?

1. _____
2. _____
3. _____

5 things I'm grateful for..

1. _____
2. _____
3. _____
4. _____
5. _____

Intentions for my sleep tonight..

1. _____
2. _____
3. _____

What do I want to do differently tomorrow?

1. _____
2. _____
3. _____

What went well today?

1. _____
2. _____
3. _____

5 things I'm grateful for..

1. _____
2. _____
3. _____
4. _____
5. _____

Intentions for my sleep tonight..

1. _____
2. _____
3. _____

What do I want to do differently tomorrow?

1. _____
2. _____
3. _____

Date __ / __ / 20__

What went well today?

1. _____
2. _____
3. _____

5 things I'm grateful for..

1. _____
2. _____
3. _____
4. _____
5. _____

Intentions for my sleep tonight..

1. _____
2. _____
3. _____

What do I want to do differently tomorrow?

1. _____
2. _____
3. _____

Date __ / __ / 20__

What went well today?

1. _____
2. _____
3. _____

5 things I'm grateful for..

1. _____
2. _____
3. _____
4. _____
5. _____

Intentions for my sleep tonight..

1. _____
2. _____
3. _____

What do I want to do differently tomorrow?

1. _____
2. _____
3. _____

Date __ / __ / 20__

What went well today?

1. _____
2. _____
3. _____

5 things I'm grateful for..

1. _____
2. _____
3. _____
4. _____
5. _____

Intentions for my sleep tonight..

1. _____
2. _____
3. _____

What do I want to do differently tomorrow?

1. _____
2. _____
3. _____

Date __ / __ / 20__

What went well today?

1. _____
2. _____
3. _____

5 things I'm grateful for..

1. _____
2. _____
3. _____
4. _____
5. _____

Intentions for my sleep tonight..

1. _____
2. _____
3. _____

What do I want to do differently tomorrow?

1. _____
2. _____
3. _____

Date __ / __ / 20__

What went well today?

1. _____
2. _____
3. _____

5 things I'm grateful for..

1. _____
2. _____
3. _____
4. _____
5. _____

Intentions for my sleep tonight..

1. _____
2. _____
3. _____

What do I want to do differently tomorrow?

1. _____
2. _____
3. _____

What went well today?

1. _____
2. _____
3. _____

5 things I'm grateful for..

1. _____
2. _____
3. _____
4. _____
5. _____

Intentions for my sleep tonight..

1. _____
2. _____
3. _____

What do I want to do differently tomorrow?

1. _____
2. _____
3. _____

Date __ / __ / 20__

What went well today?

1. _____
2. _____
3. _____

5 things I'm grateful for..

1. _____
2. _____
3. _____
4. _____
5. _____

Intentions for my sleep tonight..

1. _____
2. _____
3. _____

What do I want to do differently tomorrow?

1. _____
2. _____
3. _____

Date __ / __ / 20__

What went well today?

1. _____
2. _____
3. _____

5 things I'm grateful for..

1. _____
2. _____
3. _____
4. _____
5. _____

Intentions for my sleep tonight..

1. _____
2. _____
3. _____

What do I want to do differently tomorrow?

1. _____
2. _____
3. _____

Date __ / __ / 20__

What went well today?

1. _____
2. _____
3. _____

5 things I'm grateful for..

1. _____
2. _____
3. _____
4. _____
5. _____

Intentions for my sleep tonight..

1. _____
2. _____
3. _____

What do I want to do differently tomorrow?

1. _____
2. _____
3. _____

What went well today?

1. _____
2. _____
3. _____

5 things I'm grateful for..

1. _____
2. _____
3. _____
4. _____
5. _____

Intentions for my sleep tonight..

1. _____
2. _____
3. _____

What do I want to do differently tomorrow?

1. _____
2. _____
3. _____

What went well today?

1. _____
2. _____
3. _____

5 things I'm grateful for..

1. _____
2. _____
3. _____
4. _____
5. _____

Intentions for my sleep tonight..

1. _____
2. _____
3. _____

What do I want to do differently tomorrow?

1. _____
2. _____
3. _____

Date __ / __ / 20__

What went well today?

1. _____
2. _____
3. _____

5 things I'm grateful for..

1. _____
2. _____
3. _____
4. _____
5. _____

Intentions for my sleep tonight..

1. _____
2. _____
3. _____

What do I want to do differently tomorrow?

1. _____
2. _____
3. _____

What went well today?

1.
2.
3.

5 things I'm grateful for..

1.
2.
3.
4.
5.

Intentions for my sleep tonight..

1.
2.
3.

What do I want to do differently tomorrow?

1.
2.
3.

Date __ / __ / 20__

What went well today?

1. _____
2. _____
3. _____

5 things I'm grateful for..

1. _____
2. _____
3. _____
4. _____
5. _____

Intentions for my sleep tonight..

1. _____
2. _____
3. _____

What do I want to do differently tomorrow?

1. _____
2. _____
3. _____

What went well today?

1. _____
2. _____
3. _____

5 things I'm grateful for..

1. _____
2. _____
3. _____
4. _____
5. _____

Intentions for my sleep tonight..

1. _____
2. _____
3. _____

What do I want to do differently tomorrow?

1. _____
2. _____
3. _____

Date __ / __ / 20__

What went well today?

1. _____
2. _____
3. _____

5 things I'm grateful for..

1. _____
2. _____
3. _____
4. _____
5. _____

Intentions for my sleep tonight..

1. _____
2. _____
3. _____

What do I want to do differently tomorrow?

1. _____
2. _____
3. _____

What went well today?

1.
2.
3.

5 things I'm grateful for..

1.
2.
3.
4.
5.

Intentions for my sleep tonight..

1.
2.
3.

What do I want to do differently tomorrow?

1.
2.
3.

Date __ / __ / 20__

What went well today?

1. _____
2. _____
3. _____

5 things I'm grateful for..

1. _____
2. _____
3. _____
4. _____
5. _____

Intentions for my sleep tonight..

1. _____
2. _____
3. _____

What do I want to do differently tomorrow?

1. _____
2. _____
3. _____

Date __ / __ / 20__

What went well today?

1. _____
2. _____
3. _____

5 things I'm grateful for..

1. _____
2. _____
3. _____
4. _____
5. _____

Intentions for my sleep tonight..

1. _____
2. _____
3. _____

What do I want to do differently tomorrow?

1. _____
2. _____
3. _____

What went well today?

1. _____
2. _____
3. _____

5 things I'm grateful for..

1. _____
2. _____
3. _____
4. _____
5. _____

Intentions for my sleep tonight..

1. _____
2. _____
3. _____

What do I want to do differently tomorrow?

1. _____
2. _____
3. _____

What went well today?

1. _____
2. _____
3. _____

5 things I'm grateful for..

1. _____
2. _____
3. _____
4. _____
5. _____

Intentions for my sleep tonight..

1. _____
2. _____
3. _____

What do I want to do differently tomorrow?

1. _____
2. _____
3. _____

What went well today?

1. _____
2. _____
3. _____

5 things I'm grateful for..

1. _____
2. _____
3. _____
4. _____
5. _____

Intentions for my sleep tonight..

1. _____
2. _____
3. _____

What do I want to do differently tomorrow?

1. _____
2. _____
3. _____

Date __ / __ / 20__

What went well today?

1. _____
2. _____
3. _____

5 things I'm grateful for..

1. _____
2. _____
3. _____
4. _____
5. _____

Intentions for my sleep tonight..

1. _____
2. _____
3. _____

What do I want to do differently tomorrow?

1. _____
2. _____
3. _____

Date __ / __ / 20__

What went well today?

1. _____
2. _____
3. _____

5 things I'm grateful for..

1. _____
2. _____
3. _____
4. _____
5. _____

Intentions for my sleep tonight..

1. _____
2. _____
3. _____

What do I want to do differently tomorrow?

1. _____
2. _____
3. _____

Date __ / __ / 20__

What went well today?

1.
2.
3.

5 things I'm grateful for..

1.
2.
3.
4.
5.

Intentions for my sleep tonight..

1.
2.
3.

What do I want to do differently tomorrow?

1.
2.
3.

Date __ / __ / 20__

What went well today?

1. _____
2. _____
3. _____

5 things I'm grateful for..

1. _____
2. _____
3. _____
4. _____
5. _____

Intentions for my sleep tonight..

1. _____
2. _____
3. _____

What do I want to do differently tomorrow?

1. _____
2. _____
3. _____

What went well today?

1. _____
2. _____
3. _____

5 things I'm grateful for..

1. _____
2. _____
3. _____
4. _____
5. _____

Intentions for my sleep tonight..

1. _____
2. _____
3. _____

What do I want to do differently tomorrow?

1. _____
2. _____
3. _____

Date __ / __ / 20__

What went well today?

1. _____
2. _____
3. _____

5 things I'm grateful for..

1. _____
2. _____
3. _____
4. _____
5. _____

Intentions for my sleep tonight..

1. _____
2. _____
3. _____

What do I want to do differently tomorrow?

1. _____
2. _____
3. _____

Date __ / __ / 20__

What went well today?

1. _____
2. _____
3. _____

5 things I'm grateful for..

1. _____
2. _____
3. _____
4. _____
5. _____

Intentions for my sleep tonight..

1. _____
2. _____
3. _____

What do I want to do differently tomorrow?

1. _____
2. _____
3. _____

Date __ / __ / 20__

What went well today?

1. _____
2. _____
3. _____

5 things I'm grateful for..

1. _____
2. _____
3. _____
4. _____
5. _____

Intentions for my sleep tonight..

1. _____
2. _____
3. _____

What do I want to do differently tomorrow?

1. _____
2. _____
3. _____

What went well today?

1. _____
2. _____
3. _____

5 things I'm grateful for..

1. _____
2. _____
3. _____
4. _____
5. _____

Intentions for my sleep tonight..

1. _____
2. _____
3. _____

What do I want to do differently tomorrow?

1. _____
2. _____
3. _____

Date __ / __ / 20__

What went well today?

1.
2.
3.

5 things I'm grateful for..

1.
2.
3.
4.
5.

Intentions for my sleep tonight..

1.
2.
3.

What do I want to do differently tomorrow?

1.
2.
3.

Date ___ / ___ / 20___

What went well today?

1. _____
2. _____
3. _____

5 things I'm grateful for..

1. _____
2. _____
3. _____
4. _____
5. _____

Intentions for my sleep tonight..

1. _____
2. _____
3. _____

What do I want to do differently tomorrow?

1. _____
2. _____
3. _____

What went well today?

1. _____
2. _____
3. _____

5 things I'm grateful for..

1. _____
2. _____
3. _____
4. _____
5. _____

Intentions for my sleep tonight..

1. _____
2. _____
3. _____

What do I want to do differently tomorrow?

1. _____
2. _____
3. _____

What went well today?

1. _____
2. _____
3. _____

5 things I'm grateful for..

1. _____
2. _____
3. _____
4. _____
5. _____

Intentions for my sleep tonight..

1. _____
2. _____
3. _____

What do I want to do differently tomorrow?

1. _____
2. _____
3. _____

What went well today?

1. _____
2. _____
3. _____

5 things I'm grateful for..

1. _____
2. _____
3. _____
4. _____
5. _____

Intentions for my sleep tonight..

1. _____
2. _____
3. _____

What do I want to do differently tomorrow?

1. _____
2. _____
3. _____

Date __ / __ / 20__

What went well today?

1. _____
2. _____
3. _____

5 things I'm grateful for..

1. _____
2. _____
3. _____
4. _____
5. _____

Intentions for my sleep tonight..

1. _____
2. _____
3. _____

What do I want to do differently tomorrow?

1. _____
2. _____
3. _____

Date __ / __ / 20__

What went well today?

1. _____
2. _____
3. _____

5 things I'm grateful for..

1. _____
2. _____
3. _____
4. _____
5. _____

Intentions for my sleep tonight..

1. _____
2. _____
3. _____

What do I want to do differently tomorrow?

1. _____
2. _____
3. _____

Date __ / __ / 20__

What went well today?

1. _____
2. _____
3. _____

5 things I'm grateful for..

1. _____
2. _____
3. _____
4. _____
5. _____

Intentions for my sleep tonight..

1. _____
2. _____
3. _____

What do I want to do differently tomorrow?

1. _____
2. _____
3. _____

Date __ / __ / 20__

What went well today?

1. _____
2. _____
3. _____

5 things I'm grateful for..

1. _____
2. _____
3. _____
4. _____
5. _____

Intentions for my sleep tonight..

1. _____
2. _____
3. _____

What do I want to do differently tomorrow?

1. _____
2. _____
3. _____

What went well today?

1. _____
2. _____
3. _____

5 things I'm grateful for..

1. _____
2. _____
3. _____
4. _____
5. _____

Intentions for my sleep tonight..

1. _____
2. _____
3. _____

What do I want to do differently tomorrow?

1. _____
2. _____
3. _____

Date __ / __ / 20__

What went well today?

1. _____
2. _____
3. _____

5 things I'm grateful for..

1. _____
2. _____
3. _____
4. _____
5. _____

Intentions for my sleep tonight..

1. _____
2. _____
3. _____

What do I want to do differently tomorrow?

1. _____
2. _____
3. _____

Conscious & Calm

We hope you enjoyed using this journal and are already experiencing the benefits of a bedtime routine; a better night's sleep, more clarity and feelings of calm.

Conscious & Calm runs courses and workshops based on proven Cognitive-Behavioural strategies to help you create a life of calm, balance and fulfilment. These courses and workshops are designed to support you to improve your emotional well-being, stay more present and connected with your kids and teach your children how to do the same.

To continue on your journey of self-care and well-being, find out more here:

www.consciousandcalm.com

www.facebook.com/consciousandcalm

www.facebook.com/groups/candcmums (mums only)

www.instagram.com/conscious_and_calm

Printed in Great Britain
by Amazon

SARAH MA

The Internationals

Chatto & Windus
LONDON

500 911531

Published by Chatto & Windus 2003

2 4 6 8 10 9 7 5 3 1

Copyright © Sarah May 2003

Sarah May has asserted her right under the Copyright, Designs
and Patents Act 1988 to be identified as the author of this work

First published in Great Britain in 2003 by
Chatto & Windus
Random House, 20 Vauxhall Bridge Road,
London SW1V 2SA

Random House Australia (Pty) Limited
20 Alfred Street, Milsons Point, Sydney,
New South Wales 2061, Australia

Random House New Zealand Limited
18 Poland Road, Glenfield,
Auckland 10, New Zealand

Random House South Africa (Pty) Limited
Endulini, 5A Jubilee Road, Parktown 2193, South Africa

The Random House Group Limited Reg. No. 954009
www.randomhouse.co.uk

A CIP catalogue record for this book
is available from the British Library

ISBN 0 7011 7282 7

Papers used by Random House are natural,
recyclable products made from wood grown in sustainable forests;
the manufacturing processes conform to the environmental
regulations of the country of origin

Typeset in Monotype Bembo by
Palimpsest Book Production Limited, Polmont, Stirlingshire
Printed and bound in Great Britain by
Mackays of Chatham PLC

for G. G.

We mean to enquire whether any war is just, and then what is just in war.

Huig de Groot (Dutch jurist and statesman, 1583–1645),
De Jure Belli ac Pacis, 1625

In 1989, the Serbian Parliament revoked the autonomy granted Kosovo –
a province of Serbia – under the 1974 Socialist Federal Republic of
Yugoslavia Constitution. Resulting protests led – in July 1990 – to
Kosovo Albanians proclaiming Kosovo's independence, and adopting a
policy of non-violent resistance against Belgrade. However, when the
November 1995 Dayton Peace negotiations to end the wars of secession in
Bosnia failed to address Kosovo's status, peaceful resistance had – by 1996
– turned into armed struggle.

Between 1997 and 1998 political violence and human rights abuse
against Kosovo Albanian civilians in Kosovo by the Yugoslav authorities
steadily rose, resulting in a 200 per cent increase in the number of asylum
seekers in Europe.

The massacre of civilians at Racak in January 1999 provoked NATO
to renew its threat of air strikes against the Federal Republic of Yugoslavia.
In February, direct negotiations between FRY and Kosovo Albanian leader-
ship, under joint EU and US auspices, took place at Rambouillet, France.
In March, a second round of failed talks took place, and on 24 March, after
an ultimatum from US envoy, Richard Holbrooke, to Slobodan Milosevič
failed to persuade Belgrade to accept the proposals of the Rambouillet
agreement, NATO began air-strikes against the Federal Republic of
Yugoslavia.

Operation Allied Force lasted 78 days, and was suspended on 10 June
1999.

War was never declared and a peace agreement was never signed.

I

10°c above freezing...

25 March 1999 / The day after threatened NATO air-strikes begin on the Federal Republic of Yugoslavia

Yesterday's freak blizzard was over, temperatures were rising and there was hardly any snow left lying. At 8.30 a.m., a senator took the helicopter scheduled for Harvey Mauser from *America Worldwide*, which meant that Harvey had to wait an hour in the lobby of the Aleksandar Palace Hotel while reception tried to find another one.

Eventually, raincoat flapping, Harvey made his way over the thawing wasteland behind the hotel towards the recently completed helipad followed by Flora, his translator. The helicopter looked like something the American Coastguard had sold for scrap thirty years ago, but he climbed into it anyway. If he didn't get the figures his office needed, his life, as he knew it, would be over. Either way this piece of scrap metal held his destiny in its mangled blades.

He checked his pocket for the map they had paid some kid twelve hours' overtime to fax through, leant over and brusquely fastened Flora's seat-belt for her, then gave the pilot a light thump on the back as a signal to take off.

They were at the border in fifteen minutes.

The pilot, who modelled his dress code on American TV series no longer broadcast anywhere in the western hemisphere, and who was wearing sunspecs despite the fog creeping in, tilted the helicopter on her side and took her down.

Harvey felt a wave of nausea rush up from the pit of his ill-fed stomach.

'I'm a vertigo sufferer,' he yelled at Flora, clinging on to a strap hanging from the door. 'Tell him to straighten up.'

She leant forward and shouted something at the pilot, who laughed.

'He says it's better this way,' she said placidly.

'Tell him he'll be spending the next month scraping out the puke unless he straightens up.'

Flora took this in, staring at the back of the pilot's head. 'He says it's better this way,' she repeated.

They continued their sideways plunge out of the sky until the helicopter was low enough to hover. Harvey looked out of the window, first without, then with binoculars.

'Fifty thousand? Seventy thousand?' he said, turning to Flora.

'It's difficult to tell because of the mud. And the fog,' she added.

He looked again. She was right, it was impossible to separate people from mud and God knows what else. He instinctively put his hand to his nose thinking he could smell what he saw. There were so many bodies covering the earth that it hadn't had a chance to freeze.

'That's the army,' Flora said, pointing to the groups of men standing about in uniform.

He aimed the binoculars at them. 'Whose?'

She shrugged.

'Not many,' he said turning away from the soldiers, back to the mass of dispossessed. 'But I think', he carried on slowly, 'it's nearer sixty thousand than seventy.' He got the faxed map out of his pocket and made a quick note by the shaded block of territory on the other side of the border thinking, the smaller the country, the bigger the cause for war. 'What about the other borders? Anything happening there?'

Flora shook her head.

'You mean this is it?' he said, sounding disappointed. 'Can you get any closer?'

They jerked nearer the ground where the appearance of the helicopter was spreading panic.

Through the 8x21SP magnifying lens, Harvey saw one woman throw herself down and lie there prostrate. They buzzed around a bit more, his binoculars pressed against the window.

3

'Christ, I can't believe it. You should see this guy down here.' He gestured vaguely at the queue stretching back from the border fence along the railway track.

'What?' Flora said, trying to see.

'Jesus Christ, I just don't believe it.' He took the binoculars away from his face, rubbed his eyes then pressed them back again, even harder this time. 'He's talking on a mobile phone. They've got fucking mobiles down there.' He scanned over the mud and bodies again then sat back, shaking his head in disbelief.

'This isn't Africa,' Flora said.

The pilot mumbled something and mimed dropping a bomb.

'Yeah, yeah. Boom,' Harvey said, tired of this alien sense of humour. 'OK, OK, tell him to turn her round. I'm done.'

Flora relayed his order to the pilot. Who did a dramatic turn, rose slowly, and headed back in the direction of the Aleksandar Palace Hotel.

On the way Harvey made a mental comparison with what he had seen in Bosnia, Rwanda and elsewhere, then swiftly jotted down the numbers 3, 4, 3. On the basis that sixty thousand were being detained at the border, there would be one refugee to every eight citizens if the Republic let them in. In this context the number was impressive, but 'context' meant a lot of boring details that headline readers didn't have the time for. If only NATO could be counted on to deploy ground troops there would be more guarantee of longevity to reportage and he would be able to start using the word 'war' with assurance. He sighed and looked at the numbers he had written down.

When he got back to the hotel he had an hour to turn round in. At midday he had a private audience with the President of the Republic. He went down to reception to wait for the car they were sending. During the five minutes he had left before it was due to arrive, he had the receptionist put a call through to the United States.

'Hello, Pat? That you, Pat? It's Harvey Mauser. No, not Harvey L, Harvey M. "M" for Mauser. Yeah, right, fine, fine.' He turned his back on the receptionist, who was smirking, and fixed his attention on the flags flapping outside the window instead. He couldn't remember them being there when he arrived yesterday and nearly lost his drift. 'Hello? No, the line's OK, I'm still here, and I've got those figures you wanted.' He

4

managed, with difficulty, to get the screwed-up fax out of his trouser pocket so that he could read the numbers he'd written on the back earlier.

He crossed out the first number '3', and put a '4' down instead. 'I reckon we've got four weeks' worth of headline coverage here, maybe more,' he said down the mouthpiece. Five thousand miles away on the other end of the phone there was silence. He decided to keep it short. 'Three weeks pretty substantial filling and . . . say four weeks' worth of atrocities when they clean up afterwards. War Tribunal stuff. But that'll be sporadic. The borders here are still closed.'

Five thousand miles away there was a grunt, then the line went dead.

Harvey sat in reception, half-watching a film on the TV rigged to the wall. He couldn't remember the name of it, but knew he'd taken his daughter, Lou, to the cinema to see it. She must have been about ten at the time. *Gnome* . . . something or other. But what was the name of the cinema? He sat watching the screen and while he could bring to mind his daughter's face at the age of ten, he couldn't for the life of him remember what she looked like now.

There was no sign of the car the President's office was meant to be sending. Forty-five minutes later, hungry, he picked up the phone again.

'Hello? Pat? Could you get Pat for me? Oh all right, you'll have to give her this message then. It's Harvey Mauser. No, not Harvey L, Harvey M. "M" for Mauser,' he repeated. Lower this time so the receptionist couldn't hear. 'I gave her some figures earlier, and now I've had some time to reflect, I reckon they were a little optimistic. You got that? It's important. There's a fucking war going on out here,' he yelled, then hung up.

The receptionist, who was busy trying on a pair of ski boots he was hoping to buy off the porter, didn't look up.

Two hours after the appointed time, with Harvey clean out of Deutschmarks, having given all the notes he had on him to the receptionist to get him to call the President's office and find out what the hell was going on, the car arrived.

The President of the small Republic, somewhere in the middle of nowhere, got up early that morning. Leaving the Private Residence he passed the manicurist who had an appointment

5

with his wife, then got into the back of the presidential car next to his daughter, Elena.

They dropped Elena off at school at 8.00 a.m. The contractions in his stomach (at the sight of her receding back) died down as the driver pulled over at the butcher's to pick up a cold sausage for him. The butcher waved from behind the counter inside the shop, and the President waved back. This was something they had done for the past twenty-five years, although now he was President and had smoked-glass windows in his car, the butcher couldn't see him wave back. He relied on the butcher's wave at 8.15 a.m. every day in the same way he relied on the contractions he felt in his stomach as his daughter disappeared into the play-ground. He was old enough to know that these were the sort of things a man kept himself company with inside a prison cell.

He was half-way through the sausage by the time they stopped at the lights next to the Orthodox cathedral. A Roma boy with a cache of sparkling watches pushed a small child over to the black Mercedes as it slid to a halt. The child, who was barely four, tottered over with his bucket of water and filthy cloth and started slapping it over the car windows.

The hand and cloth moved backwards and forwards across the bottom of the glass as far up as the child could reach. The driver thumped the horn a couple of times and pressed the window switch. As all the windows in the car automatically slid down he leant across and shouted at the child to get lost. In a split second the bucket was dropped and a filthy pair of hands gripped on to the top of the back window. When half his body was inside the car the grinning child thrust his hand out into the President's face.

The President started hitting the child's head, but the tiny hand remained thrust in his face. He tried to reach the button that controlled the windows, but the driver got there before him. The child's weight was no match for the automatic window mechanism on a Mercedes and, realising this, he pushed himself back out of the car, turning his head sideways to pull it through the small gap left.

The Roma boy with the watches, now talking to a girl with flowers, had his back to them. The woman in the green *burek* stall had her attention fixed on something happening further up the boulevard. The cars behind them were revving and sounding their horns and the driver, in a sudden panic, stepped on the accelerator.

The window, still partially open, started making a clanking

sound and when they braked a few minutes later by billboards advertising Republika Foods, there was a thud against the side of the car, followed by laughter. The child was still there, hanging on. The driver was shouting and the President, outraged by this unnatural persistence, tried to prise the tiny fingers off the top of the window where they had reappeared. At last the child let go and the window shot back up into its socket.

The car was once again sealed to the outside world and sped off, after having dropped its excess weight into the middle of three lanes of accelerating traffic. The President didn't look back, and by the time they pulled up in front of the government offices, barely visible in the growing fog, he was chewing on his last mouthful of sausage.

His meeting with Janus Taylor from the EU, a prominent negotiator within the international community, had been scheduled for 9.00 a.m. At 10.00 a.m. Mr Taylor's office rang to say that, due to fog, Mr Taylor's plane had been unable to land at the Republic's airport. This was the only airport in the country; there were air sanctions to the north and west, and snow in Bulgaria. The flight had been re-directed south to Thessaloniki in Greece.

'The fog is not likely to lift today, Mr President.'

The President listened to the secretary's voice, enthralled by her precision as she described, from hundreds of miles away, the fog he was sitting in the middle of.

'Mr President?'

'Uh?'

'We are arranging to have an embassy car sent to the airport so that Mr Taylor can be driven from Thessaloniki. We hope to re-schedule the meeting for this afternoon,' she carried on smoothly. 'Between 3.00 and 3.15? I am sorry I cannot be more precise than this at the moment.'

'Well, that's a relief,' the President said.

Apart from an uncomfortable scratching sound this elicited no response.

'Mr President?' she said again, after a while. The voice was beginning to sound a fraction less sure of itself. 'I do not understand. Is this arrangement not suitable for you, sir? Unfortunately Mr Taylor has to be back in Brussels this evening so if this is not suitable, perhaps a telephone meeting would be possible. Do you have a secure line?'

'Not even to my wife.' The President let out a sudden laugh. 'I think we both know that there's no such thing as a secure line . . . unless you want to use carrier pigeons. But our neighbours take air sanctions very seriously and even birds don't make it past radar.'

Silence.

'I will inform Mr Taylor that the meeting has been re-scheduled for between 3.00 and 3.15,' she said, and put the phone down.

The President listened to the line go dead and sat back in his chair. His government's election promise of a 6.5 per cent growth in the country's GDP couldn't possibly be fulfilled now, but this wasn't why Janus Taylor, whom he had spent the last eighteen months trying to arrange a meeting with, was coming today. Janus Taylor was coming because there were an estimated 65,000 unin-vited guests on his country's border with Kosovo. The thoughts, feelings, hopes and fears of his tiny Republic were getting inter-national coverage and important ball players such as Janus Taylor were currently indulging him. Although, as his wife pointed out to him from the depths of their bed the other night, unless he had ideas of becoming a war criminal he had no hope of getting to see any Foreign Secretaries.

He made some quick notes on the sheet of paper in front of him, which was the only thing on his desk. After organising the events of his day chronologically, he usually (for his own benefit) then organised them in hierarchical order. Presented with that day's events, however, he drew a blank, and wasn't entirely con-vinced that opening the Republic's first McDonald's on national TV came bottom of the list.

He shook his head to clear it, combed his hair and, leaning over with difficulty, buffed his shoes to a shine with the sleeve of his suit jacket.

As he sat up his eye caught the Republic's seven-year-old flag, which had been cleaned and re-positioned on the wall directly behind his desk in time for today's meeting with Janus Taylor. The flag had become infamous for reducing him to tears the first time it was unveiled. He buzzed his secretary and told her to get hold of the Prime Minister.

Luka Mitrovič walked into his office an hour later. The overall effect of Luka was sleek, despite his surprising ability to switch from an attitude of complete superiority to one of utter servility. Ambition dominated his entire life and he had long since lost any sense of right and wrong.

He remained standing, not out of deference, but because this was what he always did in other people's offices.

'Ah, Luka. I want you to take the interview with Harvey Mauser from *America Worldwide* at midday.'

'Of course.'

'No statements and no promises.'

'But you're appearing on TV tonight opening our first McDonald's. That could almost amount to a declaration . . .'

'If he comments on this tell him that, speaking as one democrat to another, you think he'll understand when you say that this is a free country. We have as much right as anyone to eat Big Macs.'

'Is that our statement?'

'What?'

'That we have as much right as anyone to eat Big Macs?'

The President held tightly on to the edge of the desk.

'It's 11.45 now,' Luka added, without looking at his watch.

'I know. Send the car at 1.45.' The President finished folding the piece of paper on his desk into the smallest square possible. 'He can wait.'

Tomo woke up, his head still ringing from the Techno bar, Flux, the night before. It was 6.00 a.m., too late to go back to sleep. On the other side of the wall he could hear his parents' syncopated snoring.

The light started to touch familiar objects – mostly childhood bric-à-brac. A laptop on the desk, so sleek it was already reflecting the dull morning light, was the only thing in the room that signified anything other than a child's existence. Partly the fault of his mother, he supposed, but mostly the fault of himself.

He got out of bed and felt around the desk for his spectacles, then pulled up one squeaking set of shutters. There was washing hanging from the balcony outside just as there was washing hanging from every balcony in the wall of apartments opposite. Beyond the city he was just able to make out the hump of mountain that was the first thing he had looked at every morning since the beginning of his life. First from the crook of his mother's arms, then from an upturned orange crate and now as a man, standing on his own two feet smoking a foreign cigarette he had cajoled from an international last night. He looked at the box: Lucky Strike. He liked that.

The sign from the newly constructed Aleksandar Palace Hotel was lit. They had still only erected the first four letters and, from the twelfth floor of their high-rise, it looked as though the name ALEK had been written in neon green across the base of the mountain. He laughed a short cynical laugh at having his view of the world at dawn ruined in this way, and turned away from the window.

At 8.00 a.m. he got off the bus at the main crossroads in the city centre and headed to Dal Fufo's, the coffee bar opposite the Italian embassy. The visa queue was already stretching along the front of the building and around the corner into the thickening fog. Two policemen sat on the bonnet of their car eating breakfast and laughing together. Their laughter signified to Tomo, as policemen's laughter always did, a gloating over some gross miscarriage of justice.

He sat at one of the pavement tables under the plastic awning, still sagging in places under the weight of snow from yesterday's blizzard. The waitress was irritated at having to take an outside order and, when she eventually brought his coffee, put the cup down so forcefully that half of its contents spilt into the saucer. He drank the coffee, pushed a fifty-dinar note into the slops then made his way back through the fog to the offices Republika Foods shared with a restaurant, hairdresser's, academic press and internet company. When he got to the sixth floor the receptionist was smiling. She only ever smiled when she had bad news to impart.

'Tomo. You're late. They've started without you.' The smile broadened. 'Boris called an emergency meeting fifteen minutes ago.' She was about to add something else when the switchboard started bleeping.

'Good morning. Republika Foods,' she said brightly, then mouthed at Tomo, 'Meeting Room One.'

Sighing, he made his way up the narrow chipboard corridor past the water dispenser that was always empty, to Meeting Room One. He could hear the sound of Boris's voice coming from inside.

'This is going to be the largest initiative since we first started up in 1995.'

'What's the budget?' someone said.

'There isn't one yet, but in order to attract the sort of export contracts the government wants us to attract, it's going to have to be . . . to be big,' he concluded bravely.

Tomo knocked and entered.

Boris, who was standing by the window, turned round and gave him a quick smile.

'OK, what are we up against?'

Tomo sat down at the boardroom table where jars of hot peppers, mushrooms and Ayvar, the company's paprika sauce, were displayed along with some bright yellow sachets of powdered soup.

Boris, who used to work in then manage a shoe factory, was trying to make the best job he could of the irrevocable shift in his life from industry to commerce. His mentality, as a result, veered dangerously between that of a dethroned monarch and a small-time crook. It made him unpredictable and irrational, but also gave him a surprising ability to assess other men's worth.

Boris walked over to the whiteboard.

'OK,' he repeated, tapping a marker pen against the board, 'what are we up against?'

'Coca-Cola?' a boy called Nikko mumbled into his pad.

In two strides Boris crossed the floor to Nikko. He lifted his ex-machinist's hand and thumped him so hard on the back that the boy was sent into the surface of the table, which he clawed at, wheezing, as if it had suddenly become vertical and he was trying to hold on.

Outside, the fog shifted and sunlight started to penetrate it.

The room fell silent. Then there was a squeak as Boris started to write on the board. Nobody looked at Nikko, unable to sit up and gasping for breath.

'We need a campaign,' he announced, 'and Tomo's going to come up with the words for one. Once we have the words, you, Violetta,' he said, pointing to a young woman dressed as a Goth, who stared vaguely back at him, 'are going to come up with an image.'

Tomo, watching the sunlight shining weakly through the jars of preserved vegetables, barely heard Boris. He was focusing so hard on the preserved red chillies that they were beginning to seem unfamiliar. This used to be a favourite pastime of his during childhood. He could do the same thing with words. When he looked up, he was surprised to see his name on the whiteboard.

'You've got two weeks, the lot of you, to come up with something. Now let's get to work.'

People hurriedly pushed their chairs back and made for the door. Nikko managed to get to his feet, but couldn't stand up straight. Tomo was staring uncomprehending at his name on the board. They were all nearly at the door when Boris yelled, 'Will somebody get rid of those fucking vegetables.'

Ellen Rudinski was alone in a new house, in a new country, pouring the last of a bottle of wine into her glass. She had opened the bottle just before her husband, the new American Vice-Ambassador, phoned from the embassy. Throughout the conversation she remained calm and straightforward, giving the impression that she was in control and that he had a wife busily unpacking and piecing together a new home for them . . . that they were on the brink of a new adventure even.

The removal men, who didn't speak English, took the wrong boxes upstairs and left the wrong ones downstairs. She had probably overpaid them as well. While she was upstairs she heard them playing the piano and guessed that, if John had been there or she had been someone different, they wouldn't have dared to do that.

Before she started drinking, she had managed to locate the stereo system and one case of CDs. She tried to dance in time to Dick Powell's 'Lullaby of Broadway', but the rubber soles of her shoes got stuck on the parquet, so she just stepped in time to the music towards the kitchen and the corkscrew. On the way back into the lounge, with a second bottle of wine, she passed a mirror hung above the fireplace. Later that would be taken down – she didn't like mirrors in conspicuous places – but she took a look now because old habits die hard. She was going the same way countless other women like her went: too much make-up, far too much. In Argentina she had succumbed to cut-price plastic surgery and with this she had lost her last ounce of sophistication. She hated being alone and she hated being with people. The only person whose company she could stand was that of Peter, her brother.

'Lullaby of Broadway' came to an end and 'Pop goes your Heart' started up. Dick wouldn't have dreamt of letting any song run on for more than three minutes. Snippets of sunshine, that was all people could cope with, otherwise they got bloated and felt sick.

The wavy-haired tenor voice filled the house, spreading the word just as it had throughout the Depression when it crooned to hundreds of Busby Berkeley girls sitting at white baby grands in cinemas across the country while outside dust storms raged. And the word was that there was more to life than death. Death wasn't worth bothering about because it wasn't all that it was cut out to be. The voice, in its jingle-jangle way, reassured her that it knew this for certain.

She poured herself another glass of wine, forgetting to stop when it reached the top so that it spilt over her hands. The phone started ringing.

She picked it up.

'Ellen? Ellen, that you?'

Ellen started to laugh. Dick was going on about how to get to heaven on a mule and here was her mother-in-law whose usually thick voice was high and hysterical. She wiped her hand, still dripping with wine, on her sweatshirt.

'For God's sake, Ellen.'

'What? What is it?'

Panic broke over her. It didn't take much, and her mother-in-law brought it out in her more than anyone else.

'Is it the girls? They're all right aren't they?' Ellen said, suddenly remembering that she was a mother.

Marianna would be sixteen now and Sylvie fourteen. Their grandmother had them in New York where their education was being expensively and immaculately completed.

'The girls are fine. It's John.'

'But John's here,' Ellen insisted. He had to be; she'd seen him this morning and spoken to him on the phone. 'We just got here. He's at the embassy. Betty, I don't understand.' She stared at the skis she had started to unpack earlier, but couldn't remember the name for them or what they were used for. Her head was hurting.

'Haven't you got the TV on?' Betty said, in the same tone of voice that reprimanded her when she forgot to take her medication.

'No, no, I don't. The TV's still packed. I was listening to music, and dancing, and . . .'

'Shut up, Ellen, I don't have time for this now. I'm sitting here, thousands of miles away, watching the American embassy over there going up in flames. They're burning it down.'

Ellen had never heard Betty's voice break before, but it was breaking now. Down the line she heard the chink of her bracelets against the marble phone console.

'When did you last speak to John?'

'I don't know. Two hours ago?'

'Two hours ago?'

'Wait,' Ellen shouted, 'I'll try the other line.'

She left the receiver face-up on the floor and went running into the kitchen. John had left her an emergency number that morning, under the alphabet magnets they still carted around with them from when the children were small.

She tried the number. The lines weren't down, but nobody was picking up.

'Betty? No answer. It's OK, they have a safe room there, he's . . .'

'For God's sake keep trying and phone me as soon as you hear anything.'

The line went dead.

Dick had stopped singing.

She drained the glass of wine she was holding despite the thumping in her head, and tried to find the TV.

When she did, it was too heavy to lift out of the box so she had to cut the cardboard away from the screen and do the best she could with the aerial. Crouching on the floor she flicked through the channels until she got *America Worldwide*.

Harvey Mauser's earnest face stared out from among giant plastic toadstools in the interior of the Republic's new McDonald's.

The President stood behind him holding a hamburger and shifting its unphotogenic filling back into place while waiting for the cue to start eating.

She pressed on the controls again until, beyond the confines of satellite and cable, she found MR1, the national TV station. The camera zoomed excitedly in and out, in and out on the flames rising from cars with diplomatic plates in the embassy car park.

The gardens were full of people and the camera focused for a while on protestors still trying to scale the outside railings, but then the police arrived and started pulling them off. Reinforcements followed and soon policemen were scaling fences that before had been swarming with protestors.

The protestors inside the grounds failed to notice the increasing number of men in uniform among them. As a viewer, it was difficult to separate one faction from another. A man with a spray can got as far as NATO GO HOME before being clubbed quickly and effectively to the ground. A girl with long hair turned crazed eyes to the camera before falling to the ground in the same way. Circled, the protestors broke into chanting. A few managed to give the impression that chaos prevailed by making a run for it, but they were soon picked off the fences and kicked still.

There were flames rising from the white building her husband was inside. The collective roar of small splintering explosions and the sound of police sirens filled the room.

If she stood in one place for more than ten minutes the mud came over her boots.

She'd been shifting her weight about like this for twelve hours.

The helicopter had been and gone, she didn't know how long ago, a long time ago, and the woman who had fallen on her face in the mud still hadn't got up. A policeman had come over to tell her to shut up and one of her children tried to pull her to her feet, but they both gave up. The wailing had petered out, but she was still lying there. Every now and then Aida would look at her then look somewhere else.

All the children, as far as she could tell, had given up asking questions.

She was wearing her favourite T-shirt, with the slogan *dressed to kill* on it. Earlier there had been fog and she remembered holding on to her father's hand. You could never tell what fog brought with it or, worst of all, what it would take away when it went. All she knew was that the fog was something with an appetite. People disappeared in fog, villages disappeared; whole countries could disappear.

Days ago, a gun had been held against her head and since then time had been divided into time before the gun and time after.

There was a girl nearby whose make-up, unlike Aida's, hadn't come off yet. She'd spent the whole day reading a book in a foreign language, reached the end of it, and gone back to the beginning.

It was dark now and the border was lost to sight as was the country behind them and the country in front. For a few moments it no longer mattered whether they crossed the border or not because the border, to all intents and purposes, wasn't there.

The only thing she could be sure about was that someone somewhere knew more about all of this than she did.

12 °c

4 April 1999 / Agreement with Macedonian authorities to open border and admit refugees to NATO - built refugee camps on condition that western countries agree to take 91,000 refugees in a Humanitarian Evacuation Programme

At 8.00 a.m. the President's car made its way along the new stretch of dual carriageway in the direction of the mountains and the Hotel Vista. Also heading west and visible in the rear-view mirror was a car with the American Ambassador and new Vice-Ambassador inside. The hospitality pig-shoot had been postponed to coincide with the government's decision to open the borders. This meant that, despite the riot at the US embassy and the fact that the Ambassador couldn't get to his office now for marine snipers, the Americans had something to thank them for.

Fifteen miles out of the city the dual carriageway stopped abruptly and they hit a stretch of road that had a well-earned reputation for fatalities. Soon they were in the mountains, which had grown slowly around them. As the driver of the Americans' car manoeuvred round the boulders in the road while simultaneously negotiating hairpin bends, John Rudinski read through the list of animals it was possible to hunt at Mavro, disconcerted.

'Moufflon? What's a moufflon for Chrissake?'

'Aren't they extinct?' the Ambassador said.

The tanned Colonel, sitting up in front next to the driver, shook his head. 'It's a sheep. A mountain sheep. Guess you'd have to use a hell of a lot of cattle prongs to get any kind of sport out of sheep-hunting though.'

The road got smaller and smaller until at last the lake came into sight. The Americans took on board the fact that it was breath-taking, but kept silent. Awe and wonder weren't expected of them.

At a glance, the Hotel Vista had a whiff of Colorado about it, but this didn't make John Rudinski feel at home. It disconcerted him. In the same way the moufflon did. Higher up above the tree-line there was snow, but the slopes were a post-season brown. Despite the fact that the skiers were gone, the chairlifts were still running with a rattling emptiness that jarred on his nerves. Incongruity and contradiction made him nauseous.

The function room where the buffet breakfast was laid out – much in demand for weddings among wealthy Republicans – looked drab with only four people in it. The carpet was stained with other people's excesses and the anaemic walls failed to keep out either the smell of chlorine from the swimming pool next door or the sounds of a ghettoblaster, playing in order to conceal the sounds a large German was making as a masseur did to him what he had been overpaid to do.

The Ambassador watched Rudinski walk round the buffet table a second time, his plate still empty. Despite being given specific instructions about the pig-shoot, he had turned up at the embassy this morning in a suit.

Rudinski shifted nervously, dropping a piece of cheese on the floor.

'My daughter was with me at the embassy last week,' the Ambassador announced suddenly to the rest of the party, watching Rudinski pick the cheese up from the floor, blow the muck off it then eat it.

The Colonel stood looking out of the window, swallowing his food with difficulty. He didn't like eating, or many other bodily functions for that matter.

'During the incident,' the Ambassador clarified.

The President thought he should stop eating at this point. 'A most regrettable incident.'

'She thought she was going to die.'

The President saw himself watching Elena disappear into the playground every morning from behind his smoked-glass window, but couldn't make the connection between his feelings at that moment and those of the Ambassador, whose daughter had been at the embassy during the protest. Empathy wasn't part of a politician's education.

'We were on our way to the new McDonald's,' the Ambassador said.

The President, who wondered if he would ever get the taste of hamburger out of his mouth after that night, quickly followed this with, 'But you've seen this sort of thing before . . . you must have known it wasn't anything more than . . . than . . .'

'A student prank?'

'Exactly. A student prank.'

The Ambassador smiled slowly at him.

Aware that he'd fallen into a trap, the President turned to the Vice-Ambassador, who – he very quickly ascertained – was a nervous man, unable to look anyone in the eye. There was something of the insomniac about him, which unsettled the President, who was himself a heavy sleeper.

John Rudinski, wiping his fingers on a napkin, caught another whiff of brutality in the air – stronger this time – as the President of the Republic turned to him in his hunting jacket, stained with debris from the buffet breakfast.

Earlier, when they first arrived at the hotel, he and the President had headed for the toilets at the same time. This was the sort of thing that Rudinski, under normal circumstances, assiduously avoided, but today he was disorientated. So they stood at the urinals, Rudinski pressed so far in that his shoes hung over the open gutter and his knees dug into the tiled wall, while the President stood about a foot away, pissing loudly and with satisfaction. The pee froze in Rudinski's urinary tract as the toes of his shoes got splashed by the contents of the President's bladder, coursing along the gutter.

After the breakfast reception the party were taken in a four-wheel drive up a mountain track. The President wound down one of the windows and leant out, took a lungful of air then drew his head back in, smiling childishly. None of the Americans said anything.

'Looks like good skiing,' Rudinski said, his eyes sweeping over the mountains.

'It is,' the President replied, relieved to pick up a compliment at last.

'It's your largest resort?'

'Our only.'

'Ah. I heard there was another one somewhere along this stretch of mountains.'

'Have you ever been to a ski resort run by Albanians?'

The Colonel smiled appreciatively.

John Rudinski looked concerned. Strong opinions were one thing, but strong feelings strictly taboo.

They stopped in deep forest where the summit of the mountain was no longer visible. Rudinski shivered in his suit. The temperature at this altitude was low and the sunlight there was didn't make it through the trees to the forest floor.

The pig-run had already been set up.

The Vice-Ambassador and Ambassador were talking tersely together, trying not to raise their voices. Every now and then one of them let out a hiss.

'Does Mr Rudinski not like surprises?' the President said at last. 'Don't worry, the suspense won't last for long.'

Several minutes later a group of men bearing rifle cases emerged from a nearby van watched proudly by the President.

The Colonel leapt at them. 'Jesus,' he kept saying, turning this private armoury over and over in his hands.

John Rudinski hung in the background, terrified by the smell of blood now out in the open, and so different from the boardroom barbarism he was used to. The Colonel took him over every inch of the weapon handed him, but in the event he didn't fire a single shot.

The silence split suddenly with one of the least digestible sounds of animal fear – screaming pigs. The President, Ambassador and Colonel turned one of the pigs into pork between them while the men lit bonfires around the run.

By midday the air in that part of the forest was full of the smell of roasting pork. The three butchers, all differences forgotten, were happy; they had killed a pig and had that pig's blood on their hands. Murder was a great equaliser. Rudinski was the odd man out. They stood around the fires, the President wiping his hands on the remaining bread and using a slice of it to mop up the grease from his chin. The Colonel swallowed his last mouthful with a short sharp motion, and the Ambassador lay back among the pine needles, his hand resting on his belly.

'Mr Rudinski doesn't have much of an appetite,' the President said with a furtive glance at the figure shivering by the fire and gazing up at the sky.

'He's a Jew,' the Colonel whispered with just the corner of his mouth. 'And a vegetarian.'

They took the four-wheel drive back down the mountain to the Hotel Vista where they switched to the Ambassador's car, the President joining the Americans on the way home. The Colonel sat in front with one hand over his stomach and the other over his mouth, trying to stifle the belches he felt rising. The inside of a car was more Rudinski's natural habitat and although the President caught him sniffing at his hands for traces of the shoot, he looked better.

'So, the border's open,' Rudinski said, turning at last to the business in hand and the reason the morning had been endured.

'As long as the terms of our Agreement are honoured, yes.'

The US flag flapped on the bonnet of the car as they sped back to the city.

'And where are you going to put the refugees? What sites have been allocated for the five camps?'

The President let his chin sink severely on to his chest. This was exactly what he had been wondering himself. He stared thoughtfully out of the window.

'Or is that a state secret?' Rudinski goaded him, growing in confidence as they left the mountains and the scene of the pig slaughter behind.

The President continued to stare out of the window across what would, in the summer months, become a fertile valley. And there, between the twin minarets of a mosque, he saw a field. This field, it came slowly back to him, was the subject of much debate and nobody could determine whether it belonged to the government of the country or the Albanian Municipality. He made a split-second decision.

'There,' he said pointing, and turned round to smile at Rudinski and the Ambassador. 'The site for the first camp.'

Rudinski, taken aback, slid along the seat until he was virtually sitting on the President's lap and peered out of the window.

'Where?'

The President wound the window down.

Rudinski saw the mosque and recoiled suddenly from this vision of the east. When something flew into his eye through the open window he could almost have believed it was a grain of sand.

'There's a field beyond the mosque.'

'Where are we?'

'Stengova.'

'Stengo what?'

'Stengova. Only thirty-eight kilometres from the city centre.'

'That's where you're going to put the first one? That's official?'

The President nodded and wound the window up.

The pig's blood had gone straight to his head.

When Tomo got to Dal Fufo's that morning, Violetta from Republika Foods was sitting at the table under the awning he usually sat at. He was debating whether to join her or not, when she looked up and saw him. Pretending to be surprised, he made his way over to the table. This half an hour before work was the only time he got to himself, but Violetta was busily shunting her papers into a pile and clearing space for him. When the waitress came out to take his order, she asked for another coffee.

'So how's the copy for the campaign going?'

'It isn't,' he said.

'Same here. Look.'

She pushed a sheet of paper over the table to him.

There was a sketch of the main footbridge over the Vardar, the river that flowed through the city centre. Standing on the bridge was a group of would-be suicides waiting for the bloated corpses of some horses to be carried away by the current before jumping in themselves. Tomo laughed as she pulled the sketch back towards her.

'So, can you think of any words to go with that?'

'Life is beautiful,' he said, staring at the visa queue.

Violetta penned the words 'Life is Beautiful' across the top of her sketch.

The heavy eye make-up and deep purple lipstick were the same, but he thought he'd caught a glimmer of something beyond her usual despondency that kept everyone in the office, apart from Boris, at arm's length.

Although Tomo had written the copy for nearly all of her designs, they had never actually collaborated on a campaign. If the words he came up with were any good, the next time he saw them was on the finished proofs. If they were bad, they ended up back on his desk, crossed through.

She smoothed her hand over the drawing.

'I think I'll go with this life is beautiful thing.' She paused. 'All

22

we need is some product placement. What would stop this group of suicides from jumping?'

'A jar of pickled mushrooms?'

'What would stop you from jumping?' she asked suddenly, then, without waiting for an answer, she signalled to the waitress.

'I'll get these,' Tomo said quickly.

'I don't want the bill, I want a raki.'

He didn't know whether to stay and watch what was obviously part of a ritual or to make his excuses and go.

She drank it without satisfaction, breathing out with relief when the glass was empty. Her lips left a heavy purple stain on the shot glass.

'We went to the same school,' Tomo said after a while.

This time she did call for the bill.

'You were a couple of years above me. I remember now.'

He waited for her to acknowledge this, but she didn't and before he knew it the bill was paid and they were walking along the pavement away from Dal Fufo's.

'Sorry, I said I'd pay.'

'Don't worry about it. You spent more than ten minutes in my company. That's something I should pay for.'

He wanted to say something to counteract this, but couldn't think of anything.

They walked in silence to the building Republika had its offices in. There was a removal van parked in the bay outside, surrounded by a group of Roma trying to help carry the furniture piled on the pavement.

'Where's all this going?' Tomo asked.

'Floor Five.'

'Who's moving in?'

The desks, chairs, filing cabinets and computers were all new.

'World Refugee Council.'

Tomo and Violetta walked into the lobby. A woman stood thumping on the 'call lift' button.

'What's wrong with this thing?' she said in English.

At last the lift arrived and she walked impatiently into the back of it followed by a small woman wearing huge earrings.

'Floor Five,' she said.

Violetta leant forward and pressed the button for Floor Six. Neither of the women noticed.

23

'What's your apartment like?'

'A shoebox,' the one with the earrings said.

'Mine too.' The other one sighed and leant her head back. 'At least you've got a cleaner.'

'There's not exactly much to clean.'

The lift stopped with a jolt and the women moved forward, pressing up against the doors waiting for them to open.

They rattled apart with a sporadic ringing sound.

'This is Floor Six,' Violetta said as the reception for Republika Foods came into view.

'But we need Five.'

The women ran back into the lift as the doors jerked shut.

'You see what happens when they agree to open the borders,' Tomo said.

Violetta shook her head. 'They've been here for weeks. Lying low, waiting for this moment.'

Later that morning Tomo went down to Kibo, the restaurant on the fourth floor, but there wasn't a table free.

'We're full,' one of the waitresses shouted.

'I just wanted omelette.'

'And where are you going to eat this omelette? We've got no tables left, no chairs, and no plates. Look, even my pad's run out. I've got nothing but an armful of orders.' Angry, she thrust her arm in his face. Items from Kibo's encylopaedic menu were scrawled over her flesh from wrist to armpit. 'Satisfied?'

The driver opened the door and Ellen Rudinski got out of the car in the way she had been taught to thirty years ago, with both legs together in order to minimise the chances of putting one's crotch on display. Her heel got caught in the door and she would have ended up in the gutter if the driver hadn't caught her by the elbow.

The British Ambassador's wife, Anne Hargreaves, was interested enough in this small scene to stop and introduce herself.

Ellen straightened up. The two women shook hands. She recognised Anne Hargreaves from the shoulders up, having spotted her trimming the hedge that separated their two residences.

'Heading for the International Wives Club meeting?' the British Ambassador's wife asked.

Ellen nodded.

Anne Hargreaves laughed.

They fell into step.

'You should have let me know. My driver could have brought us both,' Ellen said, managing to drag up some vestige of her former sophistication.

'Don't worry. I always take the bus.'

A lot of British wives Ellen had met over the years had this strange obsession with patronising public transport. Acquiring pointless hobbies and overcoming unnecessary obstacles seemed to be a national trait.

'I heard your husband got caught in the embassy riot.'

'Didn't turn out to be much of a riot.'

They cut across the main square.

'This gives you some idea of what the city used to look like before the earthquake. Notice the formality – a formality entirely without grandeur. I mean, you wouldn't exactly travel miles to see this, would you?'

'They have earthquakes here?'

'The one in the sixties destroyed most of the Ottoman city.'

Ellen looked at the old cream and yellow buildings, and tried to achieve some sense of past glory, but failed. She detected an underlying attachment to the city in Anne Hargreaves.

They stopped outside a small bookshop and the British Ambassador's wife disappeared inside. She came out a few minutes later pushing a book into her bag. Ellen caught the name 'Donne' and recognised it from a chapter in John's book of quotations that he used for speech writing.

They reached the city's largest shopping mall. This wasn't unlike a multistorey car park, its sides open to the elements so that in the winter months the corridors of shops became wind tunnels and, during blizzards, snow banked up in large obstructive drifts. The coffee shop that was their destination, one of the less depressing ones in this half-deserted retail palace, was on the second storey.

'We're late,' Anne whispered, pushing open the frosted-glass door. 'The President's wife is giving a speech.'

They crept past the banquettes covered in fake pink leather and sat down at the first table they could. There was a small Union Jack on a plastic stand in the centre of the table. The women sitting round it smiled at Anne and stared at Ellen.

'It will take time for us to understand each other, but please do take the time. We are a proud and hopeful country, but more than 320,000 of us are unemployed.'

Coughing broke out from a sofa in the corner where a woman with dyed blonde hair, holding a miniature Russian flag in her hands, had lit up. Her cheeks shook as she coughed.

'Economically we're still recovering from the Greek embargo in 1994 when we were cut off from our trading port of Thessaloniki as well as overland routes through the Federal Republic of Yugoslavia because of UN sanctions.' Irina Yupović paused. 'These aren't things you recover from overnight.'

There were murmurs in the room and a clattering from behind the counter as the smell of coffee rose.

Ellen sensed resentment towards the President's wife for her inappropriate comments and for not making them laugh.

'We have constantly rubbed shoulders with war.'

A thin grey woman sitting at a table with the Austrian flag on it tutted audibly.

'Now we are 70 per cent down on export contracts and transport costs are up by 30 per cent. Trade and investment agreements have been postponed and are likely to be cancelled. This is where we're at.'

She smiled, and her voice betrayed no emotion.

'So, please just give us a bit of time. I know that our intentions are the same and that together we can see this crisis through.'

The Austrian stood up, but the President's wife hadn't finished.

'Society is never perfect – it consists of more than one person.'

For the sake of all the international wives gathered there, the Austrian broke into a frantic round of applause in order to bring the speech to an end. Soon all the women were clapping.

The President's wife, confused, picked up her briefcase and shook hands with the Austrian.

The waiters started to bring pots of coffee over to the tables.

A baby belonging to a pathologically glamorous young Mexican woman started to cry. The women on her table huddled round it, having decided that it was the President's wife's fault the baby was now in tears.

'Ladies, can I have your attention, please.'

It was the Austrian, desperate to get the coffee morning back on to its usual footing.

'I think we can turn to more mundane matters now. So let's start with this T-shirt.'

She pulled the one she was wearing out from her chest and Ellen made out a globe surrounded by the slogan 'International Wives Care'.

'These are now for sale, thanks to the efforts of Joanna Harris.'

Joanna Harris blushed and was applauded.

'Other things on our agenda this morning are the forthcoming tour of Roman ruins in the south of the Republic, and . . .' she held her hand up for silence, pausing, '. . . a shopping trip to the hypermarket-sized M&S in Thessaloniki.'

There was light-hearted cheering as the overweight treasurer, at a signal from the Austrian, started to make her way through the crowds of women with a clipboard, taking down names for the shopping and archaeology trips.

'Ladies, we always have fun,' she reminded them severely. 'So step forward and sign your name over to the clipboard.'

For a few moments, listening to the President's wife, Ellen felt that she was somewhere rather than nowhere. Now that feeling was gone. She tried to hold on to some memory of it, but couldn't. The President's wife was gone, having left without anyone noticing.

Anne Hargreaves had also vanished.

The woman opposite her leant over the table.

'Excuse me, are you English?'

Ellen laughed. 'No.'

'Ah.' The woman sat back and exchanged glances with the other women round the table. 'It's just that this is the English table.' Her hand went out for the plastic Union Jack and she started twirling it between thumb and forefinger. 'You're American, aren't you? The American table's just over there.'

Ellen stood up stupidly, obediently, and started walking towards the table with the American flag on it then changed her mind and headed for the door instead.

Behind her someone called out her name, but she ignored it.

Once outside she walked over to the wall in the middle of the walkway, looking over the parapet to the shopping mall's lower level. From her vantage point she was able to see a man she recognised coming out of the chemist's.

Leaning as far over as she could, she yelled, 'Peter!'

Her brother turned and looked up at her, his hand across his eyes because of the sunlight.

'Ellen? That you?'

'Up here.'

He took his hand away.

'Why didn't you say you were coming?' she shouted down. 'I thought you weren't due until next week.'

'I just flew in from New York yesterday,' he shouted back. 'Wait there. I'm coming up.'

In a rush of excitement she ran along the walkway to the top of the stairs and waited by the chess club for him to appear.

A couple of minutes later he was there and Ellen Rudinski collapsed with relief into him.

'The World Refugee Council got wind two days ago of the government's announcement to open the borders, so I came early.'

'Of course.' Ellen vaguely remembered this information rising up through the miasma of morning television. 'You want a drink? There's a bar up by the cinema. I passed it earlier.'

She caught hold of his hand and led the way back past the coffee shop to the far end of the mall.

The bar, done out in original and not retro sixties style, was open.

'I can't believe you're here,' Ellen said as they both instinctively sat down at the table furthest from the door.

'You knew I'd show up sooner or later,' he said.

The waiter brought a whisky and a beer.

Ellen watched her brother drink.

There existed between them the closeness of siblings who have shared an unhappy childhood. They knew each other's history inside out. She knew that his right eye drooped slightly because of a run-in with Kenyan police in Nairobi over a young boy he had stupidly given his heart to. He was beaten so badly that his face never did regain its symmetry. The beating terrified him but not to the point of annihilating his suicidal aptitude for love. Peter could love anyone and anything – even those two policemen.

Falling in love stupidly, tragically, was a pattern he was committed to. It happened again when he was working for an NGO in Albania, but this time there was no beating.

'How are the girls?'

'I don't know. I haven't spoken to them. I think John speaks to them. He phones from the embassy.'

'But doesn't tell you?'

She shook her head. 'It's a conspiracy between him and his mother.'

'Ellen.'

There it was, that terrible understanding and sympathy.

She put her hand out and gently stroked his arm, feeling under her fingertips the scars inflicted from a decade of heroin abuse.

'I mustn't care that much or I'd be doing something about it. Fighting them. Getting on a plane. The truth is, Peter, I don't know if I want to see the girls any more, and they certainly don't want to see me. I write to them when I'm drunk, and make the mistake of posting the letters when I'm sober. God knows what I say. I can't remember afterwards.'

'You're their mother.'

She laughed.

'That's very fetching, Peter, but in the free market it amounts to just about nothing. They'll be fine. Life's short.'

'Life is short,' he agreed.

'So you're living in town?'

'Only until the end of the week. When the camps are given sites, I'll live there.'

'You'll be within driving distance,' she said, more to herself than him. 'You want to get some lunch?'

'No, I've got to go.'

'Already?'

'I've got a meeting.' He finished the beer.

'When will I see you again?'

'Soon.'

They stood up and he hugged her. She felt her handbag slide off her lap on to her feet.

'When soon?'

'I don't know, Ellen.'

'Before you leave the city?'

'Probably not.'

'You've ruined my day showing up here like this.'

He hugged her again and made for the door.

'I'll order another ten of these once you've gone.'

She loved exposing herself like this to him. Putting the worst she could come up with on display.

'Make it a good one,' he said lightly, stepping over the threshold.

29

Kicking the handbag under the table she ran to the door.

'Peter, are you happy?'

'I'm always happy. See you around.'

He started off up the walkway, glancing at the man pasting up new posters outside the cinema.

'Peter.'

She made a lunge for him. She couldn't do nonchalance any more. These days she needed reassurance and other more concrete things.

'I love you.'

'Love you too.'

He gave an infuriating wave, the same sort he might give to anyone, and disappeared down some stairs leading to the lower level. She thought about running after him, making him commit to a date for a future meeting so that she had this to hold on to first thing in the morning and last thing at night. But the thought of the barman's eyes when she went back in to retrieve her handbag stopped her.

She had enough sense of self-preservation left for this.

Enver, the Mayor of the Municipality of Stengova, was watching television. The children had been cleared out of the room and only his father sat muttering in the corner, a pack of cards in his hand. Enver's wife put her head round the door to see if they wanted more coffee, but he waved her away.

The TV screen could hardly be seen there was so much cigarette smoke in the room. He wiped his eyes and strained forwards, certain he saw something familiar flicker across the screen. There it was again, no doubt about it. He was looking at his own house, the one he was sitting in right then. There were his children, and there were the builders up on the third floor. He watched, fascinated, as the camera swept round the outside of the house then across the disputed, uncultivated field in front of it. The voice of the Republic's President begged his people to have faith in him.

Enver's father didn't look up from his cards. The cigarette wedged in his mouth had been smoked down to a stub and the sleeves of his jacket were covered in ash. His game of Patience came out. Letting out a hoarse 'ha', he put the cigarette stub carefully in the ash-tray and glanced up at the TV screen.

'They're building a camp in our field,' he announced.

'Who is?' Enver said, stupefied.

'The English, the Americans, the Germans . . . others . . . everyone.' His father made smacking noises with his lips, an old man's habit. 'Don't mind the English,' he mumbled to himself. 'Churchill . . . Churchill . . .' he stared down at the game of Patience, '. . . was a great man.'

Enver didn't reply, he got up and went to the windows, pulling back armfuls of net curtain in order to get a look outside, but the wall surrounding their property was too high. He thought he heard lorries.

'Government gave them the field,' the old man said, watching his son's back.

Enver stood silently by the window, thinking.

Six months ago, an environmental group had turned up and spent a fortnight talking about asbestos deposits in the air from the old copper mine. There had even been some free medical checks that the entire village had turned up for, disappointed that free medication didn't come with the free examination. A team of American mining experts turned up when the environmentalists departed, and somebody started a rumour that they were going to open the mine again. Men of all ages started turning up there every morning looking for work, but the team only stayed three days before relocating up to a gold mine in Kosovo.

He started to holler. Hollering was something he did when a lot of elements came together in his mind at once. His youngest son put his head round the door first, nervously wrapping his prayer beads round his wrist.

'Get Spatim to round up all the people in the village who speak English and bring them to my office.'

The boy ran off.

When his wife appeared he shouted at her to fetch his big black overcoat.

The coat was put on and he made his way to the shoe rack by the front door. They had only started building the house two years ago, but it was already beginning to match, in proportion, the Hotel Vista in Mavro. Three families from Kosovo were living in the unfinished upper two storeys. They had managed to cross the border in February, arriving at Stengova in the middle of the night.

The echoes from Enver's last bout of hollering died down and

31

a group of children appeared on the cement steps. He kissed one at random on the forehead then left the house, crossing the short space of forecourt between front door and minibus, his mayoral vehicle. By the time he got into it his shoes and the bottom of his coat were covered in mud.

Shortly after this his wife emerged from the house, headscarf flapping and carrying a case under her arm. Enver spread his hands out on his knees as, up to her ankles in mud, she started taking gold rings out of the case and pushing them on to his fingers.

Next his older son appeared bearing an alabaster eagle painted gold, which he put into the passenger seat of the minibus. The six children tailing him carried the second mayoral eagle between them.

Enver's cousin, Balon, who had been born simple in the head, opened the huge gates in the wall that surrounded the property. Balon was not only Enver's gatekeeper but caretaker of all public buildings in the village including the mosque and the old cinema. The old cinema had once, briefly, been a shoe factory, and families with young daughters often woke to find boxes of ladies' shoes outside their gates. These offerings of Balon's were never talked about. He hauled the gates open, pulling them through the mud with severe concentration, as if history depended on him.

The main village street ran along the outside wall of the property and on the other side of this road was the field.

There were already three lorries with the insignias of national and cable TV stations on them parked in the field. It was getting dark and a group of men in bright anoraks holding torches swung round as the gates to the mayor's compound opened and the minibus reversed into the road.

Most of the men from the village were there. The crowd parted to let the minibus through then turned to follow it as it drove eight hundred yards up the village street before stopping outside Petri's restaurant. Mud, and Enver's need as Mayor to make an impression, rendered the two-minute journey by minibus necessary.

Enver made his way through the restaurant and the smell of roasting chicken to his chambers of office at the back of the building. Two men struggled behind him with the mayoral eagles and were instructed to place them on either side of the desk so that, sitting down in his black overcoat, he was flanked by the golden birds.

A few minutes later there was a knock at the door and his youngest son walked in, still fiddling nervously with his beads. Four people followed him into the office: Spatim, whose father was in prison for second-degree murder; Kushtrim, the English professor at the school; Fatos, a young actor recently returned from Albania; and Valbona, a young woman who had just completed a degree in English.

TVs went on in Stengova at dawn and weren't turned off until well after sundown. They now had access twenty-four hours a day to the rest of the world. Everyone knew why they had been called to Enver's chambers of office.

Spatim, with his father behind bars and his eldest brother on a building site in Switzerland, was responsible for his entire family and unable to join the KLA guerrillas in the mountains. He harboured this and many other dangerous regrets, but was a favourite of the Mayor.

'We need to talk business now, not politics,' Enver warned him fondly. 'They're building a camp in our field.'

Spatim slumped sullenly back in the chair. 'Politics is business with these people, nothing more.'

Petri came in with a tray of coffees and handed them round.

The English professor quoted something appropriate from his own, never published, Albanian translation of *Julius Caesar*.

Enver pressed swiftly on.

'The camp will generate a lot of revenue. These internationals will need places to live, food to eat.' He paused. 'Entertainment.'

Fatos, the young actor, leant forward, excited.

'I saw a wonderful Ray Cooney farce in Tirana,' he said. 'We could stage that here.'

Enver, who had been thinking of entertainment more in keeping with his own frequent trips to Bulgaria, wondered what on earth Fatos had spent his time in Tirana doing, then remembered that he had published a large volume of love poetry. He sighed.

'Something good is going to come of all this,' he continued.

'Computers,' Valbona said brightly. 'For the school.' This had been a fruitless but persistent campaign of hers for the past nine months.

'Maybe,' Enver conceded, 'but, more importantly, we have roads that need tarmac surfacing and a long way to go with facilities for electricity . . . these people can help us . . .' He broke into a cough, his mind wandering as it often did to a small badly furnished bed-sit in Sofia. This camp meant that he might just have enough of a reason to bring the small badly furnished woman who lived there here to Stengova without raising too much suspicion. 'You will, all of you, offer your services as translators.'

The three young people and the professor nodded.

'These internationals who are coming here to Stengova, they only have their souls to think of. The copper mines are dead . . . the shoe factory is closed. We have much more to think of. There is something at stake here for us.' He stood up, impressed with himself. 'It isn't our fault the days of honest toil are over.'

The Mayor's last comment confused everyone, including the Mayor. Uneasy at the way in which morality had crept in, he called the meeting to an end.

Fatos opened the door and the smell of roasting chicken once more accosted them.

The professor opened and closed his mouth a few times in silent preparation for a closing speech.

The Mayor, spotting this, quickly ushered them out of his chambers.

They drifted back through the half-empty restaurant under the impression that they had all taken vows, but without being really sure what it was they had bound themselves to.

Enver buttoned up his coat.

His youngest son stared proudly at him.

'You want me to carry the eagles back to the minibus?'

'No,' Enver said absently, 'no, I don't want you to do that. I want you to go home and tell your mother that I'm going to Bulgaria. I'll be back first thing tomorrow morning. Think you can remember that?'

The boy nodded.

'I'll be back first thing tomorrow morning,' he repeated. 'Oh, and tell her that it was Petri who sent me to Bulgaria. That's important. She'll understand then.'

The boy gave him a podgy smile.

'*Did* Petri tell you to go to Bulgaria?'

'Of course. I wouldn't say it otherwise, would I?'

Enver took a last look round his chambers of office then shut the door. He tidied his hair in the mirror above the bar then left the restaurant, wondering if he had enough time to drive into Kulov and buy the girl waiting for him in the bed-sit in Sofia the body spray she liked so much.

The car park at the Aleksandar Palace Hotel was full and the night air resounded to multilingual threats and curses as well as the universal blare of car horns. Since the official declaration that the borders were open, issued that morning, internationals had been falling out of the sky.

Those in the know came prepared. Windows were wound down and money changed hands. In this frenzied climate of bribery, prior reservations meant nothing. Those pious enough to feel outrage soon realised that outrage was impotent without a roof over its head.

There weren't enough rooms to be had, taxis to be hailed, servers to deal with e-mail connections, satellite dishes to accept mobile signals, or, it turned out as Harvey joined the queue, revolving doors into the hotel. In the face of this logistical log-jam the night descended into screaming chaos.

Flora, sitting in reception, saw Harvey standing in the queue outside the hotel, but it was another ten minutes before he pushed his way through the revolving doors. She stood up and started to make her way over to him across the piles of suitcases covering the floor.

Harvey tried to reach the receptionist, whose purple dickey bow was lopsided, to see if there were any messages for him.

Pat had made no allusion to him missing the riot at the embassy, and that was bad news. He shouldn't have missed it – five years ago he would have smelt it out. It wouldn't be long now before they cut his expenses account. Then he'd be asked to pay his own airfare home – it had been known to happen before – and he never could forget the sight of Todd Hunt leaving *America Worldwide* offices. Two months after that, Todd's wife had left him. That's what happened to people: they broke, and then those they loved left, in order not to get broken themselves.

He was almost at reception when Flora tapped him on the shoulder.

The sight of Flora irritated him right then.

'What is it? Are we meant to be meeting now?'

She shook her head.

'Well, it would be helpful if we could stick to the schedule, and helpful if you were less keen.'

'I need to talk to you.'

'About what?'

They were both shouting to be heard.

'Can we talk somewhere else?'

'Here's fine.'

Harvey made a point of looking around him, impatient.

'I thought I might try and get work in the camps.'

'You work for me.'

'But the pay will be better in the camps.'

'You're contracted to work for *America Worldwide*.'

'Contracted?'

'The contract. That piece of paper you were so happy to sign.'

'But . . .' Flora shrugged.

'A contract is a legally binding document. D'you understand that? This is something you've got to get the hang of . . . commitment and responsibility.'

She blew her nose.

'There was no contract. We don't have a contract.'

Harvey stared at her. She might be right. He couldn't remember a contract either.

'So what? You came all the way out here from the city to threaten me with the withdrawal of your services?'

Flora, not fully understanding, smiled. 'I like working for you, Harvey, but the camps will pay well. Better.'

They were continually buffeted against each other by the mass of internationals. Her hair went up his nose and he sneezed, grabbing hold of the top of her arm.

'You see all these people?' he said hoarsely. 'Well, half of them are here looking for work. Just like you that day. Only now I don't have enough hands to count them on. They all speak Albanian, Macedonian, English. You're common currency. In market terms more currency means less value and honey you're devaluing by the second. I could fire you and hire a new translator without moving from the spot.'

She looked at him, unsure whether he meant to do this now.

'You might get work in the camps, but then again you might not. What's the average monthly salary in this hole? Three hundred Deutschmarks? Four hundred? You aren't in a position to

36

negotiate and you certainly aren't in a position to threaten. The only thing you're in a position to do is pray that I keep paying you.'

Harvey became aware that people standing close by were staring at them. He looked down. Flora wasn't crying so much as weeping.

Carefully he let go of her arm, repulsed and fascinated. He had never reduced a woman to tears before.

He realised that he needed to get her out of reception.

'You want a drink?'

She nodded her head but made no attempt to stop crying and was still crying as she climbed up onto the bar stool.

Harvey ordered two vodkas.

The never-ending tears disconcerted him. They made him feel suddenly responsible for her. He drank his vodka, but she didn't touch hers.

'You're not Muslim, are you?'

The tears were easing off. She shook her head. 'My family's Catholic.'

'So what's wrong with the vodka?'

'I'm underage.'

Harvey didn't know what to say. His mother once told him that an honest man has no charm. This was true.

He swallowed and ordered himself another.

'So what do you want to drink?'

'Coca-Cola,' she mumbled, without looking at him.

She sipped at her drink and took a packet of cigarettes out of her pocket.

'So what's your story?' he asked her.

Her story was that she didn't have many of the Deutschmarks her father gave her left rolled up in that pair of tights in her drawer.

She hadn't been sad to see the back of her cousin's car sliding off through the slush on the road they had just come down that day in January. Afraid, but only in a way that added to her excitement; she'd flirted her way through the ranks of uniformed men at border control before passing with surprising ease into the Republic. Only to find herself looking down a similar stretch of slush-covered road with the same colour sky above it. She stood there until she couldn't feel her feet any more, a young woman with a suitcase in a foreign land, waiting for a taxi to take her to the big city.

Her mother had spent days looking for tears that never came. She had been more excited about what clothes to take, and didn't even bother to hide her disgust at the suitcase her mother dragged up out of the cellar with the faltering words, 'Your father and I took this case on our honeymoon.' It was simply snatched out of her arms, and had so many shoes and clothes packed into it that the old catch broke and a belt had to be used to keep it together. She blamed the suitcase for the fact that the taxi driver demanded to see her Deutschmarks up front before agreeing to take her to the city. Her hands shook for the first time since leaving home as she counted the money out in front of his flat eyes, watching her from inside the car with his elbow hanging out of the window, while she stood shivering in falling snow that was fast becoming a blizzard.

Her story was that every night she dialled the house in Priština that she'd lived in all her life, but the line was always dead. The last she heard her parents were hiding in the basement of their house, but that was three weeks ago. When her mother made one of those death-bed speeches that people on the edge make, touching raw nerve after raw nerve regardless of the listener's stamina.

'I came here to the city because my friend promised me a job in door-to-door make-up sales for New Flame, the Swedish company. It never materialised. Then I heard that I would be able to pick up something at the Alek, which was supposed to be flooded with internationals and only half-built so I came here and sat in reception every day for two weeks. The few I found the courage to approach either already had translators or were wary of my lack of qualifications.'

She blew smoke out through a smile.

'You were the only one to approach me.'

'I'd seen you sitting alone in reception watching the same movie over and over again.'

Flora tucked her hair behind her ears, studying herself in the mirror behind the bar then turned on him suddenly.

'That's my story. What's yours?'

Harvey didn't know what to say. It was so long since anyone had expressed any interest in him.

His entire childhood passed briefly through his mind: a myopic land without poverty or wealth, hopes or fears. A land without heroes. He could hear the sound of the sprinkler now as it hissed its way through Sunday after Sunday, and almost expected to turn round on the bar stool and see a stretch of lawn behind him.

Then there was Val; then there was Harvey and Val; then there was Harvey, Val and Lou. He would have liked to carry on, but Val had no intention of it. At some point in their life together, she started to make it clear that she had made sacrifices in order to marry him, and the more he listened to the ever-increasing list of sacrifices, the more undeserving of her he believed himself to be. Finally it got to the stage where every time he got home at night and put his keys in the lock, he expected some genie to descend from the skies and carry the whole of 1001 Lake Drive away with him, into the night, laughing.

Harvey had realised, only recently, that the main difference between Val and him was that she took everything for granted and he took nothing. He knew all these things about her, but most of all he knew that he still loved her. He loved her despite her making him feel small, despite her making him feel like an inconsequential father, and despite the fact that she didn't love him any more, and probably never had done.

'You're thinking about your wife,' Flora said.

He stared wearily at her, but didn't answer.

'Are your parents still alive?' she asked.

'No. They're dead.' He drained his glass, feeling that this didn't quite do them justice. 'They were always faithful to each other,' he added, still thinking about Val.

Later, he put Flora into a taxi outside the hotel and paid the driver the fare up front.

'I need you . . .' he started to shout through the window.

She nodded and smiled.

The taxi pulled slowly away, trying to avoid other taxis dropping off more passengers and more luggage.

'I mean I need you tomorrow morning. Tomorrow morning at 10 o'clock.'

He banged on the window but the taxi slid out from under the palms of his hands.

He made his way unsteadily up to his room. Now worth its weight in gold. He turned the shower on and had just got one shoe off when the telephone started to ring.

39

'Hello?'

'A call for you.'

'Who is it?' Reception rang off without answering and he was connected to his wife on the other side of the world.

'Harvey?'

In a second Val's voice stripped the hotel décor away. He could hear the sound of the fridge door at 1001 Lake Drive opening and shutting, and a TV in the background.

'How are you?' he asked.

'OK. Yeah, OK.'

'How's Lou?'

'Out. On a date.'

'What's he like?'

'Who?'

'The date.'

'Oh, the date. He arrived in an Alfa Romeo something or other.'

'And how was Lou?'

'She wore red. I told her not to but she wore red.'

'But how was she?'

'The red made her come up all pink. I had to tell her.' Val yawned. 'She swore at me, I hit her, then she cried.'

Harvey's heart went out momentarily to his daughter.

'She still wore red though.'

Val stopped talking. This was something she often did when she realised that she wasn't talking about herself.

'So?'

'So what?'

'Am I allowed to ask the big one.'

'The big what?'

'The big question.'

'Jesus, Harvey, you sound like you're about to propose to me or something.'

'Is she in love?'

'She isn't even eighteen yet.'

He watched steam from the hot shower drift out of the bathroom and, thinking about Todd Hunt, wondered if there was enough unbreakable stuff between Val and him to suffer the indignity, shame, humiliation and financial insecurity of him getting laid off.

'We were eighteen.'

'Were we?' She sounded unconvinced.

Five minutes later the line between them both went dead.

15°c

18 April 1999 / UN estimates that approximately half a million
Kosovo Albanians have become refugees

David Everett woke with a start to find himself on a Swiss Air
flight from Zürich, lying in a black leather seat he had tilted earlier to 'recline'. His book, *An Atlas of the Crusades*, was still open on
his lap.

He asked an air hostess called Anya for a bottle of water and a
half-bottle of champagne, both of which were brought to him
with a snarl. The hostesses they put on Balkan flights were the
ones who didn't quite make the grade. The emotionally pockmarked who had, at one time or another during their airborne
career, 'flipped': threatened passengers with the jagged edge of a
broken glass, dropped food on to laps, or shaken crying children
into comas. He could tell from the way Anya did her make-up
that she was a potential homicide.

The young man next to him eyed the bottle of champagne in
the way somebody who used to rely on the stuff but has since got
over it might eye a bottle. These were the sorts of things David
saw: the world as it was in all its unabridged reality. Sometimes
against his will. The older he became, the more he felt the weight
of it. He sighed and looked down at the book open in his neighbour's lap where there was a picture of an animal with bicycle
wheels for legs.

The man followed his gaze then hurriedly shut the book. 'I'm

42

trying to educate myself,' he apologised. 'Well, actually my girl-friend's trying to educate me. She's an art student.'

David watched as he tried to give what he thought was a frank smile, then moved his chair to the upright position.

'I'm not an art student,' the man reassured him. 'I used to be an estate agent. A very successful one,' he added, unable to completely drop the salesman's patter.

'So what are you doing now? Backpacking around the world in search of your lost soul?'

David poured the yellow liquid into the plastic beaker. His former irritation slipped away from him as he started to drink.

'No, no.' The man hesitated. 'I just felt that I wanted to do some . . . some . . .' He looked out of the window, but there was nothing there apart from acres of sky and a blinding sun.

'You wanted to do some good – find something or someone worth dying for? Don't be embarrassed, it's a widespread malady. Just look around you. You're among fellow sufferers.'

David ordered another bottle of champagne, which Anya threw at him from the aisle.

'Come on. I'm sorry. What's the name?'

'Guy,' the man said, sulkily. 'Guy Spiers.'

'David Everett.' They didn't shake hands. 'So, where are you going?'

'The Republic. I want to try and pick up some voluntary work in one of the camps.'

'How long do you plan to stay?'

'Two months. Initially.'

'Well, two months isn't long enough for you to become a true international, like most of the people on this plane,' David said, screwing his head round again and briefly taking in all fellow-passengers. 'Let me tell you now, in case you hear otherwise . . . an international is someone who loses his home through choice, and whose experience is meant to be valid to those who have lost their homes, or worse, against their will.'

'What are you, recently divorced or something?' Guy said, listening to him in horror.

'No. A journalist.'

'Look, even though I've got no idea what this place is . . .'

'It's Godforsaken,' David cut in. 'Why else would we be going there.'

He rapped the *Atlas of the Crusades* with his knuckles, and fell into another alcoholic doze.

When he came to, the seat-belt signs were flashing, and he heard Anya's grating voice over the intercom. Due to fog at the Republic's airport they wouldn't be able to land and were diverting the flight to Vienna.

'Will passengers please make their way to the Swiss Air Information Desk on landing, where you will be able to get transfer vouchers for MacAir, who are still operating a flight to the Republic today.' Anya's voice paused. 'Despite fog.'

The intercom crackled and went dead.

'The flight's cancelled,' Guy said, seeing that David was awake.

David looked out of the window. 'It can't be. We're on it.' His head and mouth felt swollen. Down below he saw the steel chimneys rising from the factories on the outskirts of Vienna.

'Does this happen often?' Guy asked.

'Not surprisingly – yes – the valley they built the country's main airport in is a meteorological phenomenon – filled with fog all year round.'

A flight's worth of hysterical internationals landed at Vienna airport half an hour later. Contrary to instructions given, they didn't just approach Swiss Air staff, but anyone in a uniform. Even baggage handlers and Customs officials were assaulted by their outrage. There was no regard for age or gender, and an elderly woman at the magazine stall was nearly knocked senseless by an Indian businessman looking for directions to the Swiss Air Information Desk.

By the time David arrived, anxiously shadowed by ex-estate agent Guy Spiers, the desk could hardly be seen.

All regard for human life was trashed within seconds in the attempt to get hold of MacAir transfer vouchers. A Spanish diplomat's family was trodden underfoot. Some Catholics from Chicago were yelling that they'd already been on a long-haul flight before changing planes at Zürich. A cross-eyed Englishman from Crown Cars, doing transport logistics for NGOs based in the Republic, managed to get his MacAir voucher first even though it meant bludgeoning a baby's head with the corner of his brief-case. People were waving blue UN passports and a young couple who had fallen asleep in each other's arms on the plane tried to explain to an air hostess that they were going to miss the girl's father's funeral. The air hostess ignored them, disgusted by their naïvety in assuming that a father's funeral would hold any sway in the world of delayed and cancelled flights.

Eventually David got his voucher and made his way to the MacAir desk where everyone from the flight was tensely waiting for Check-In to open. There were sheepish smiles of recognition born of a shared fate, and a feeling that their forbearance in these adverse circumstances deserved some official acknowledgment.

When a female member of MacAir staff finally arrived someone tried to initiate clapping, but her spitting-on-graves smile soon deterred this. Once she sat down the orderly queue became a crush of internationals, at pains to let it be known that they weren't going to have plans to save their souls thwarted by third-world levels of bureaucratic chaos. The cross-eyed Crown Cars man turned out to be a professional queue jumper, a sign in David's book that at some stage in his life he would be willing to take a child's place in a lifeboat. The Catholics from Chicago made a re-appearance, closely tailed by a pack of inebriated Hungarians, keen to make the Americans their in-flight sport.

They boarded the plane via the rear, something the older passengers remembered doing in the sixties and seventies. The Check-In process turned out to be a fantastic charade because, once on board, there was no seat allocation. There was also, more importantly, no first class.

The internationals were consumed once more by outrage. They were so outraged that they failed to notice the plane taking off until they were shunted, *en masse*, into their unallocated seats where they grappled wildly for seat-belts that didn't exist. The take-off didn't last for long. Somewhere just above tree level the pilot straightened up, and they stayed at that height for the rest of the flight, weaving in and out of the mountains. The cabin crew, consisting of one man and one woman, soon lit cigarettes, and the man pompously drew shut some blue curtains at the front of the plane. Fifteen minutes later the woman re-emerged pushing a trolley. Food was flung into laps and the trolley abandoned at the rear end of the plane for the rest of the journey, rendering the WC unusable. Just before landing, as the plane started to tilt, the trolley coursed back down the aisle of its own accord. A split second before it went crashing through the blue curtains and into the pilot's cabin, a hand emerged, checked its course, and dragged it once more behind the scenes.

The plane landed badly on the Republic's runway. The Spanish diplomat's children started screaming and crying, only to be pacified as they glided past the tanks and jeeps of the American K-For base that ran alongside it.

They emerged, as they had entered, out of the plane's rear end. The surrounding countryside, as far as the eye could see, looked as though it had been painted in camouflage.

'A new city. New adventures,' David heard the Spanish diplomat murmur to his wife, whose face must have been a picture of desolation to have provoked such desperate optimism.

The internationals clambered warily out of the plane. Fate had decreed that they should arrive alive, and for now this was enough. The fury and outrage of Vienna had been left in the west. Many of the men and women emerging under the Republic's spring skies were in charge of budgets totalling more than the country's GNP.

The sun rose on Stengova.

Bulldozers levelling land had already started work in the southern section of Stengova camp. It hadn't rained for days and a cloud of dust hung over the machines as they worked, covering families nearby still strewn across plastic sheeting.

Aida finished folding her and her father's blankets then sat back down again and looked around the tarpaulin square. In front of her were rows of tents, and behind her more tarpaulin squares. These didn't interest her, but the tents did. The tents signified something.

She opened the scuffed vanity case beside her and started to unpack it, taking out various tubes of mascara, lipsticks and other cosmetics, and laying them out in the order she had devised when they first arrived at the camp. Her eyes gave the line-up a quick professional scan: everything was present and in order.

Ten minutes later, she packed everything away. This was essential. If the make-up stayed out of the case for too long it would not only become covered in dust, it would lose its particular smell. It was also important that her father remained unaware of this morning ritual she indulged in.

When all the make-up was put away she checked to see that the book on astronomy was there, in the side pocket where she

46

kept it. After some hesitation she laid this out briefly on the tarpaulin then flicked open the pages, smelt them, and put the book away. The smelling of the pages was another part of the ritual. Every morning she had to do this to make sure that they smelt the same. The last person to read it was someone who had worn a strong perfume and who had passed their wrists across the page as they turned it.

She remembered her mother getting the vanity case out of the cupboard once a year, in order to perform the annual ceremony of making her face up to commemorate the day she met her – Aida's – father. This was the only time Aida remembered her mother forgetting to hate her life on the farmstead; the only time she stopped talking about mud and talked instead – even if only for a couple of hours – about pavements, and the kind of shoes it was possible to wear when walking on them. After her mother's death, she inherited the vanity case. For her mother it had signified a promise broken, and for herself, a promise as yet unfulfilled.

Aida felt that the make-up and the book, brought out into daylight every morning, amounted to more than her sum total and that they somehow made the tarpaulin square inviolable.

Temperatures were high for April and she watched the internationals moving about in T-shirts and shorts that had been eagerly donned. She looked out for Nadia, the short Italian girl who wore a different outfit every day, and who had once interrupted her during her laying-out ceremony. Aida had expected Nadia to be impressed, but she wasn't, and in her confusion Aida had stupidly told her about the gun that had been pressed against her head on the day they were forced to leave their house. The gun seemed to impress the Italian and, since the woman was one of the few internationals who spoke Albanian, Aida had been prepared to listen to her account of watching the Albanian coastline as a child, from Italy, and how she used to wonder why there was no electricity in the country across the sea. For as long as she could remember, she had wanted to see the place that stayed dark when everywhere else was light.

Aida wasn't particularly interested in the lack of electricity in Hoxha's Albania, but then neither, it transpired, was Nadia, who had been using this as a means of getting to the point, and the point was the gun. The Italian wanted to know, more than anything, about the gun that had been riveted to Aida's head when

47

she and her father were forced to leave their home. Maybe this preoccupation with violence was something all the internationals shared.

Every time Nadia saw her she wanted to know again about the gun, and the more she tried to appropriate it, the more jealous Aida became of it. Now she was on her guard and kept a lookout at all times for this international with her strange dissolute greed for information about the gun, something that unsettled her far more than the gun itself had.

There was no sign of her so far this morning.

Aida shifted uncomfortably, her stomach aching with constipation caused by the successive ready meals as well as a lack of locks on the few toilets there were. Her bowels seized up now at the sight of the stacked yellow containers, and it wasn't safe to use the toilets late at night when there were less people. More privacy meant less safety.

She wondered briefly where her father was, then went back to staring at the rows of tents in front of her. In a tent she would be able to take her T-shirt off and wash it.

Dust from the bulldozers blew through the open flap of the vaccination tent, irritating the eyes and nerves of those who had been injecting small quantities of German measles and Vitamin A into the arms of 700 children an hour, for the past three hours. Most of them having only completed their two-day training programme yesterday.

A crowd of children who had already been vaccinated hung around inspecting the small patches of puckered skin on their arms with excitement, and watching those still waiting to be done.

Donatella, from the Italian NGO Women Against War, had tried to clear them out of the way three times already, but she didn't have a way with children and they kept coming back.

She blew the dust off her watch.

'I'm going to take an early lunch,' she said to the young girl standing next to her.

The girl, tired, nodded and misjudged the needle's entry into a boy's arm.

The boy screamed and went running out of the tent.

Donatella methodically made a note of the child's name and

tent number on the recall list and handed the girl a packet with a new syringe in it, then left.

Outside, the growing breeze was full of the pervading smell of excrement. For a few days they had managed to reach the standard for collective latrines of one per twenty people, but now they were back up to a figure of one hundred per latrine.

Making her way to the camp's main entrance, where another Italian NGO had set up a makeshift staff canteen, she somehow managed to stride and stoop at the same time. Her movements suggested that she had, at some point in her life, discarded the pursuit of happiness. She lived off her nerves, not her emotions, seeking to understand situations that were beyond the moral comprehension of most people. This was her quest. A quest that had made her – over the years – gaunt and sunken.

A different person, or even the same person brought up in a different way, might have found the round green mountains covered in forest and rising up over the valley beautiful. But she walked through the camp oblivious to the mountains, seeing only what lay directly around her, with no need of respite.

She believed in basic human need and desire, but not the myth of civilisation. People needed food, shelter, water and sanitation. Each other. They needed not to die. Take the walls of any city down and this was what you would find.

People required a minimum of five litres of water a day and there should be access to one water tap for between 200 to 250 people. Water consumption should contain less than ten faecal coliforms per 100ml, and water should be disinfected to contain between 0.3 and 0.5mg of residual chlorine per litre. If there wasn't time for collective latrines to be constructed, trenches had to be dug, and there needed to be one latrine trench for 50 to 100 people. An average ration of Kcal 2,100 per person per day was also required. These were the facts of survival. Endurance lay just beyond survival, and endurance required sheets, towels, underwear . . . condoms.

In Malawi, she was the only non-medical aid worker dealing with solid waste control to point out that a separate pit should be dug for anatomical waste. Word of this got out and she was then officially appointed to oversee disposal of the dead. Responsible in good times for the building of the cemetery, and in bad – during cholera and typhus epidemics – for the collection and disinfection of corpses and the digging of communal graves. She understood catastrophe . . . events people and countries weren't able to insure themselves against, and the work made her happy; far happier than she'd ever been in Rome.

She queued up for her bowl of stew and wished they sold beer. The more she thought about the cold beer she wasn't drinking, the more she wanted it.

Peter Miller from the World Refugee Council caught up with her in the queue.

'Are you going to the meeting?' she asked.

He nodded. 'Have you seen Spatim anywhere?'

'Spatim? No. Not since this morning. Looking for Nadia's a good alternative to looking for Spatim – they seem to spend a lot of their time together.'

'Donatella,' someone shouted.

She turned round and waited impatiently for Howard from Oxfam to join them.

'We're back down to one latrine per hundred again,' she said as they all sat down.

'I know, I know.' Howard was silent, shoving in mouthful after mouthful of stew until the bowl was empty. 'The British Tommies are good, but you have to supervise the digging or it doesn't get done. I still haven't worked out who the hell's in charge of them.'

'What about the Germans?'

'The Germans are great, but reluctant to do anything that doesn't involve using tanks.'

'Volunteers?' Peter asked.

'The best I've got is Bernardo, an ex-jacuzzi-salesman from Barcelona.'

'We have to get back up to the standard for collective latrines of one per twenty.'

'That's going to be difficult given that Oxfam haven't even been able to get water mains access today.'

'Why not, for God's sake?' Donatella said, giving in to a sudden gnawing weariness.

'Some engineers from a private French company claim that granting Oxfam access to the water mains will jeopardise fulfilment of their contract.'

'Who hired them?'

Howard shrugged and they all fell silent.

Last night twenty-five buses had arrived, with eighty people on each one. Donatella had had four hours' sleep, and she was on to her third packet of cigarettes.

'We've got to do something about that arc lamp,' she said, thinking out loud. Howard and Peter Miller automatically nodded, seeing again what had become a nightly scene: bus after bus arriving and people stepping off into light broader than daylight. They'd had to erect a fence around the arrival point to stop people running away out of sheer confusion. Or fear. And all the women in the camp would hear the buses arriving in the middle of the night and come running up to the fences, clamouring against them looking for relatives, husbands – children they'd lost – trying to get to them.

'I can't think of an alternative,' Howard said. 'There are hardly any streetlights and we need to get some sort of registration process underway immediately because otherwise . . .'

'Why do the buses always arrive in the middle of the night?' Peter said suddenly.

Howard was about to answer when a man came walking towards them, a crying woman following close behind him. People stopped what they were doing to stare, and a group of children running up the field with a car tyre stopped in their tracks as well.

It was Howard the man wanted, approaching him with the palms of his hands upturned. Half-way through his rant he started to raise his voice, and the woman behind him left off tugging at his elbows in order to cover her face with her hands she was crying so heavily.

Howard listened and tried to calm the man, saying something that seemed to satisfy him. The creases in his face dropped out, and he took hold of Howard's hand, stroking it several times. Then he walked away, leaving the woman behind. She wasn't crying as heavily as she had been, but she was still crying. She tried to take hold of Howard's hands as the man had done, but he gently prised them off, turning his back on her with a shrug.

She carried on pleading with all of them in turn, especially Donatella, until Howard said something final to her and she turned and walked away in the wake of her husband.

'What was that?' Donatella asked.

'Headache material,' Howard said through a cigarette. 'The man

51

has two wives. He gets a visa through for him and the old woman to go to America with the children, but he doesn't want to because he doesn't want to leave his other younger wife behind. So . . . he gives the visa to the older wife and tells her to take the children to America on her own. Him and the young wife will join her when they can. You saw, she doesn't want to go. She thinks the young wife should go to America with the children. Now nobody wants the visa; nobody wants to go to America.'

'So?'

'I put myself in his shoes. The old wife's taking the visa, and has to go to America with the children tomorrow. She tried to sell me the visa but I told her it's no good, she has to go. The man's happy, the woman's unhappy. I'm going to find Marcus – see you at the meeting later,' he finished, getting up and plodding off in the direction of the Médecins Sans Frontières tent.

'Howard speaks good Albanian,' Peter said.

'He didn't two months ago – he's a natural linguist.'

'How many languages does he speak?'

'About twelve. The more you learn, the easier it becomes, apparently. He says you can tell what a country looks like, even if you've never been there before, from the language.'

They watched Donatella's colleague, Nadia, her face streaked with sweat as she ran around the tents frantically looking for trau-matised children.

The boys rolling the car tyre with a stick went running down the hill. Within seconds Nadia was giving chase, yelling something in Italian after them. They yelped back, a series of whoops as uni-versal as they were incoherent.

Once in his chambers of office, Enver sat down, rubbed his eyes and sighed. The morning sun started to filter through the blinds, exposing the dust on the desk and the mayoral eagles. He wiped his hand across their static feathers, waiting for the two men to arrive. Men whose names his brother gave him last night on the phone and told him to trust.

The Municipality of Stengova was relatively wealthy – largely due to the efforts of his brother, Emshi, now living in New York. A lot of new building work, including Enver's own home, was subsidised by the trade in arms that passed through the small caravan parked outside Emshi's house in Queens.

Following his brother's relocation to the United States five years ago, Enver had been made Mayor of Stengova. Had since become, in fact, nothing more than Emshi by proxy. None of this bothered him much, until one morning recently, when he came across his younger son pushing a yellow NYC taxi around the hallway under the impression that Uncle Emshi still drove one. The sight had inexplicably bothered Enver who, next to his son's serious play, felt suddenly childish.

He heard the kitchen door bang followed, a few minutes later, by the shuffle of feet on the backstairs to his office. The door opened and Petri walked in, an apron already on under his anorak. Enver got irritably to his feet and walked over to a cabinet in the corner of the room.

'Sorry I'm late,' Petri said, his mouth going loose as it always did when he apologised.

Enver shrugged and poured himself, slowly and methodically, a glass of Johnnie Walker.

'I had to mend my daughter's stereo. I didn't get time last night, and I promised her . . . I promised her.'

Ignoring him, Enver suddenly tipped up his head and drained the glass, then walked back to his desk and sat down, the empty glass still in his hand.

'You know what they're like. Daughters.'

'Bring me three coffees.'

Petri hesitated a second then nodded and left the room.

He'd only been gone two minutes when the two men walked in.

Enver started at their arrival and its unnecessary silence, making it malicious in his mind. The lack of warning, of shutting doors and footsteps on the stairs, set him on edge.

'Benny Schmalz,' the first man said, extending his hand for Enver to shake. He started to cough then sat down in the nearest chair. The second man – more of a boy – sat down immediately afterwards without waiting to be asked.

Enver recognised Benny. He'd seen him around Stengova, and even here in Petri's. He had a face with overgenerous features that looked as though they had been put to no good use. Especially the mouth. The 'Schmalz' was a hangover from the days in Germany when the Albanian had tried – unsuccessfully – to set up his own building supplies business. Emshi liked unsuccessful people

53

because of the quick knowledge of human nature a run of bad luck could give a person. He knew how to work with them . . . how to make them work for him.

'Did anybody see you leave the camp?'

Benny shook his head.

'The German and British soldiers are still trying to erect security fences around the camp. There aren't enough Republican policemen to patrol a perimeter that doesn't exist, and so . . .' He shrugged. 'Human traffic in and out of the camp is regular. No,' he added, 'we weren't seen.'

Enver breathed out more heavily than he had meant to. He saw the man's eyes flicker over him and the empty whisky glass he had placed on the desk only minutes before.

Apart from what was useful for their purpose, the only thing Emshi had told him about Benny Schmalz was that he had survived successive solitary confinements. Enver didn't find this hard to believe. He also guessed that he was somebody who held those who feared him and those who admired him in equal contempt. There was something tainted about him that men who have socially unacceptable desires can't conceal.

The young boy sitting next to him was the sole survivor of an ambush of KLA operatives by Serb soldiers in the mountains four months ago. On the summit of the mountain he had left, among other things, the girl he loved, lying face-down in the snow.

Enver watched as a slight sneer crossed the boy's face – something that had been happening sporadically since he entered the room.

He pitied the boy his bad luck in falling prey to Benny Schmalz, and was willing to overlook the sneers and swagger that implied he was a lesser being for never having followed a track of bloodied footprints in the snow, or left a beloved body, unburied, on the summit of a mountain.

'You know why you're here?' Enver said at last.

'Do *you* know why we're here?' Benny responded, with a smile.

Petri entered with a tray of coffee. The boy took his and asked for a Coca-Cola as well. This irritated Enver, but he signalled to Petri to fetch one.

'Emshi's had word that agents from the Republic's Information Bureau are here in Stengova . . .' Enver said after Petri had left.

'He has had word,' Benny said, still smiling. 'From me.'

Enver breathed in the heavy smell of coffee that filled the small room, but it didn't reassure him. '. . . Searching for arms – under cover as Republican policemen.'

There was silence in the room. Outside they could hear Petri's slow tread on the stairs as he made his way back up with the Coca-Cola.

'It's not cold,' the boy said, feeling the glass.

Nobody said anything.

'It's not cold,' he mumbled, shrugging it off.

Petri left; the same slow plod audible as he went back downstairs.

'What do you want us to do?' Benny said, suddenly. 'Me and the boy, we can't just get rid of all the policemen here.'

'No,' Enver said slowly. 'We need to make an issue of their presence. After all, it must be distressing to the people in the camp who were detained by them at the border. The internationals working here must be made to see that; must be made to recollect their treatment of the refugees, so well documented by the world's media.'

'We need the people in the camp to insist on the removal of all Republican policemen,' Benny said. 'They must be replaced by ethnic Albanian ones.'

Moving his legs apart, he hung his elbows over his knees and let his head drop forwards.

'How?' Enver asked, staring straight at him.

'We need to incite a riot,' Benny said decisively.

'How?' Enver asked again.

'The policemen at the border, they beat us,' the boy interrupted, his eyes wide. 'They were crazy. Shouting and stuff.'

Benny had been staring at his hands, but now he looked up at Enver. 'That's how,' he finished, smiling.

'But you weren't at the border on that particular occasion. You only got here three days ago,' Enver reminded him. 'Neither of you is an actual refugee – you're KLA.'

The boy stared at the eagle on the right-hand side of the desk and didn't reply.

'That's not the point,' Benny said placidly. 'He himself wasn't at the border, but someone else was. Someone who maybe isn't able to tell their story, so the boy tells it for them. Absorbs it. Say only half the people here were trapped at the border in March and maltreated by Republican policemen – you make their experience contagious so that the other half forget that they were never there. You incite their memory to recollect an event that never took place for them personally. You heard the boy,' Benny said with a quick look at him. 'That's what he's doing.'

'Their guns were jumping in their arms,' the boy added, on cue.

'I don't want guns here today,' Enver said quickly. 'Emshi doesn't want guns.'

They sat in silence again for a while after this. Emshi's long-distance orders triggered off different cravings in all of them, but none of them questioned his authority. They were, all of them, Enver thought, willing cellmates in Emshi's panopticon.

The silence was broken as the boy got suddenly to his feet, tugging his shirt out of his trousers and shouting, 'The policemen at the border beat us.'

Benny tried to pull him back into his seat, but the boy yanked himself out of his grasp.

'Look. Broken ribs,' he yelled, caught up in a frenzy of past injustices he hadn't even been party to.

'Save it for later,' Benny muttered, then shrugged again with a gesture towards the boy. He knew where the fundamental spring lay coiled in any given person, in any given situation. 'After all,' he pursued, 'what is a riot? An overheated conversation. Nothing more.'

'An overheated conversation,' Enver repeated. 'The only problem with overheated conversations is . . . that it's very difficult to determine an outcome.'

'Very difficult,' Benny agreed, and waited.

Enver glanced down at the other man's trousers, which were at least a size too big, purple, and shiny at the knees.

Benny, in his turn, took in the empty whisky glass again; the chocolate boxes with the singer – Lori's – face on them, tacked to the wall and the mayoral eagles, flanking the desk.

The boy, who had gone suddenly limp, was tucking his shirt morosely back into his trousers.

'When?' Enver asked, his face troubled.

Benny Schmalz got to his feet.

'This afternoon, that's when. There's a meeting for all international staff here in the restaurant.'

'Does that give you enough time?'

Benny shrugged. 'Have you been in the camp?'

Enver nodded and the two men shook hands. 'This afternoon, then.' He shook hands with the boy as well, whose hands were cold.

When the door shut he cleared the two chairs back against the wall then sank heavily into his own chair. The three empty coffee cups, and one Coca-Cola glass, were still lined up along the far edge of his desk. Suddenly filled with anger he leant forward and swept them on to the floor.

It took over two hours to get through passport control despite the frantic waving of UN passports. Once through, a human barricade of Roma boys selling placards of Casio watches had to be traversed before reaching the taxi rank.

David stood in the queue watching Guy, who hadn't made it through, get forced into some business transaction involving cigarette lighters and dollars. Once the Roma moved on, Guy checked to see that all his luggage was there, and nervously tried to get a flame from the lighter he'd just bought.

After twenty minutes Guy still hadn't moved from his spot outside the front of the airport.

David let out a loud whistle and waved him over. He saw the boy hesitate before gathering up his luggage and breaking into a lumbering sort of run towards the taxi rank full of Yugos.

'Extra passengers and extra baggage cost,' the taxi driver mumbled from behind huge wraparound sunspecs with lenses like puddles of petrol.

The taxis behind started leaning on their horns.

'You'll get your money,' David said.

He pushed Guy into the back of the cab where he was soon obscured by his luggage.

The taxi screeched unevenly out of the airport car park and on to the main road into the city.

'How much money have you got?' David asked.

'Lots,' Guy said. Then, after a pause, 'Is lots enough?'

David told the driver to take them to the Aleksandar Palace Hotel.

'This looks like a conference centre I once went to in Birmingham,' Guy said as they pulled into the hotel forecourt, not sure whether this made him relieved or disappointed.

This time last year the Aleksandar Palace hadn't even existed because the kind of guest willing to pay five-star rates didn't exist. The hotel had literally risen out of the dust to have its entrance obscured by four-wheel drives with UN plates and its glass façade filled with reflections of the flags of foreign nations.

'This'll cost you, but it's the best place to pick up work. I'll call you,' David added, watching the boy pull at his luggage.

'Aren't you staying here as well?'

'No – I've got somewhere else to go.'

'Wait,' Guy said as the Yugo crunched back into gear.

David wound the window down.

'Do they speak English here?' He gestured vaguely at the steel-and-glass edifice of the hotel, and the sky above.

'The whole world speaks English,' David said as the cab pulled away.

'OK, where to now?' the driver asked.

'Ulida Odredi.'

'There's no hotels on Ulida Odredi.'

'I'm staying with a friend.'

They hit a bad patch of road, full of potholes from winter's frosts and snow, and the plastic Virgin Mary, attached by a spring coil to the dashboard, jumped into life.

The driver nodded and smiled.

'What's her name?'

'Sophia.'

'That's a good name. That name makes me happy,' he said, grinning indulgently at his unexpected generosity.

'I haven't seen her for five years.'

The driver had nothing to say to this, and turned his attention to assiduously jumping lights as if his tip depended on it.

They drove into the city past the American embassy. Since last month's riot at the commencement of NATO's bombing campaign, an imposing security fence had been erected around the circumference of the building, but as far as David could see there were still more stray dogs than US marines.

They drove through the city centre past the new McDonald's, towards a stretch of tower blocks that could have been transplanted from any western council estate.

The taxi soon turned into Ulida Odredi whose strip of tarmac separated the nineteenth century from the twentieth. Tower blocks on the left-hand side of the street faced tiny squat pre-earthquake villas on the right, some of them with wells still in the front gardens.

Despite the initial drabness of the apartment blocks, on closer inspection it was possible to discern south-facing balconies and, hanging from them, strings of red peppers hung out to dry by elderly inhabitants. When the wind blew down from Mount Vodna around the high-rises the rustling sounded like a chorus of whispers. David remembered one old man whose entire kitchen was outside on his balcony. Whatever the weather, he could be seen in front of his cooker stirring various soups or stews, and the steam rising in huge billows from his balcony on frost-bitten mornings was enough to melt the snow on the balconies above.

David paid his fare plus extras and got slowly out of the taxi, craning his neck and counting the layers of apartments in the block until he got to Floor Eleven where Sophia and her mother lived. Behind him the taxi pulled noisily away and the sound of boys playing basketball rose from beyond a row of garages. Picking up his bags, he walked up the steps and into the lobby.

The dark wood and tiled interior of Petri's absorbed the smoke and conversation as well as it could. This was the first time since the camp opened that all the international staff had been gathered under one roof. Every booth was full, and there were people perched on the end of tables whose heads kept hitting the orange glass lamps hanging low and intimate. It gave the meeting a clan-destine air that Chris Woods from World in Crisis, the organisa-tion responsible for overall camp management, might have found exciting two decades ago.

Enver, Spatim and three other men sat at a table on the upstairs balcony looking out over the restaurant floor as bottles of beer were delivered to all tables by the fleet of Bulgarian waitresses.

Chris Woods, refugee camp veteran, stood up and waited with his hands in his pockets for the room to fall silent.

'Welcome to Stengova,' he said at last.

Somebody let out a loud whoop – a cry taken up by the rest of the room.

'My name's Chris Woods. I'm an Australian from Melbourne, and,' he paused, 'I'm in charge here.'

He glanced up at the Mayor's table on the balcony and waited for noise in the room to die down.

'OK, where's Howard? Howard? I'm not going to make you stand up – just raise your hand. OK – there's Howard. He's British and he works for Oxfam. I want you all to remember him because he's a phenomenon. He's the man who brings water.'

There was another round of applause.

Howard stared warily at the table in front of him.

'Some of you, I know – I've worked with before. Others, I don't – haven't. But you all need to know the following because communication here is already bad. I won't have information treated like private property – it's public property and belongs to all of us. Information isn't power – it's a dead-weight. Get rid of it or you'll sink.'

He paused.

The room breathed.

People took a few sips from the beers they'd been nursing during the speech.

'Our number-one concern is water and sanitation. You've all smelt the increasing lack of toilet facilities . . . the weather is getting and will only get hotter . . . frustration is rising and the possibility of disease-outbreak is high. Stengova camp currently houses an unhealthy population of around thirty thousand and numbers aren't likely to stop until we reach our allocated quota of fifty thousand. This is not Disneyland.'

He looked down at his fingertips, pressing them into the table edge.

'Tonight, over four thousand people will be sleeping out on plastic thanks to UNHCR.' He broke off. 'Where's UNHCR?'

A table near the window briefly raised their hands.

Chris Woods took a good long look at them.

'. . . Who gave us pipeline figures instead of in-country figures for one hundred thousand tents, which means that no one ordered any more. Dan Hale – you know who you are. This is a disaster. A very real disaster.'

There was a rumble from the UNHCR table, but it didn't amount to anything

'To those of you working with children – especially unaccompanied minors – I want to say a few quick words.

'I have no children of my own and, despite having been one

60

myself, understand little about them. However, I do know this much, and it's always proven more than enough: you cannot enter the head of a five-year-old child who's been separated – sometimes violently – from its parents. You will never be that child. What you can do is use your skills and experience to make that child a happier child. UNICEF's doing a brilliant job with its registration and family reunification programme – long may it last.'

The room waited while he drained the glass of Coca-Cola on the table in front of him.

Low conversation could be heard coming from the Mayor's balcony.

'How are we doing on relief items?'

'We're waiting for sheets, towels, underwear, eating sets . . . hats,' a young Austrian girl listed. 'And there's going to be a problem with shade soon. It's getting hotter. We're also out of condoms,' she added.

'Already?' Chris asked.

'We need to talk about the proposal for a mobile paediatric and gynaecological unit,' an American woman started shouting.

'Why does the unit have to be mobile?'

'So it can work in the village as well as the camp. Maybe other villages.'

'We need to talk about this, Genevieve,' Chris warned her.

'Well, let's talk now.'

'This is a logistics meeting. Let's try and stick to the agenda.'

'There could be people reproducing right now as we speak, there could be . . .'

The sound of a chair scraping across the balcony drowned out her rising hysteria and, the next minute, the Mayor started shouting something in Albanian at the crowd gathered in the restaurant below. Spatim, who had hold of his arm, was trying to pull him back into his seat.

'Is there some sort of problem up there?' Chris Woods yelled.

'I'm trying to translate for the Mayor,' Spatim yelled back. 'He's confusing contraception with sterilisation.'

'For Christ's sake.' The Australian let his head fall on to his chest.

Suddenly there was a thud as the body of a man fell against the outside of the restaurant window. In the lull that followed, the monotonous jabbering and muttering of a crowd stirring itself

61

into motion could be heard in the distance. Nobody moved. The next minute a young MSF doctor appeared bent double in the open doorway, his hands on his knees, and blood from a wound to the head dripping on to the wooden floor.

'Marcus?' Donatella said, getting to her feet.

The Norwegian tried to stand up straight, but couldn't.

'The camp,' he said heavily. 'A riot's broken out.'

The lull continued for a second longer, then broke.

Marcus was slammed into an upright position by the force of the internationals crowding through the doorway, only to be confronted by a wall of boxed Yamaha keyboards that had been left on the terrace earlier and were destined for the youth tent. The young doctor temporarily lost consciousness and slumped inconveniently across the threshold of Petri's restaurant. The last person to leave their dusty boot prints on Marcus's prostrate body was a young financier from Action Food Campaign.

Spatim dropped the Mayor's arms and went running out after the internationals, avoiding Marcus but stumbling over the blocks of polystyrene juddering in the wind, and sleek black electronic keyboards that had spilt out of the wrecked cardboard boxes strewn across the terrace.

Enver held on to the sticky wooden balustrade running around the balcony and waited.

Mobiles were dragged out of pockets and yanked off belt-clips in wild authoritative gestures. Nobody knew what was going on. Those who had forgotten to charge their phones muffled the cries of shame their bodies betrayed them into making.

With their heads all turned in the same direction, towards the camp gates, and their lips moving, they looked as if they were speaking in tongues. A couple of the more senior internationals had satellite phones and, around these chosen few, a hallowed space was cleared.

Chris Woods, who hadn't left Petri's with the rest, sat with his back against the wall and waited. Just like the Mayor of Stengova, six feet above him. He watched Marcus, the young MSF doctor, as he came to, lumbered on to all fours and crawled slowly along the terrace in front of the restaurant window.

Chris's hand went out for the satellite phone on the table in front of him then stopped as he heard the shuffling of feet on the balcony above his head, followed by the noise of heavy footsteps walking down the stairs, which stopped when Spatim came running back into the restaurant.

'There's a riot in the camp,' he said loudly, breathing heavily between words. 'They're rioting.'

Enver plodded to the foot of the stairs. 'They want the Republican police force removed.'

Spatim stared at him. 'I don't know – I couldn't make anything out. There was just this shouting, this . . .'

'I'm not asking you, I'm telling you,' Enver cut in, impatiently.

'You knew?' Spatim shouted, trying to come rapidly to terms with the fact that what he had taken for spontaneous action was in fact premeditated. He was about to say something else when he made out the figure of Chris Woods sitting at the table under the stairs, the soft luminous green from the digits on the satellite phone dully illuminating his face.

Enver walked over to where Spatim was standing and peered at Chris Woods.

The two men stared at each other.

They had met once before to discuss drainage and the village's water supply. The man had spoken in English and Spatim had translated.

Outside in the street, a group of men had broken away from the rest and were making their way towards the restaurant.

Petri came running out from behind the bar, towards the front door, slamming it shut. The yells of the crowd became immediately more distant as he fumbled with the various bolts of his security system.

'Don't bother – they're not trying to get in,' Chris Woods said.

Petri stood up straight and watched through the door as two men started dragging the Yamaha keyboards along the terrace.

Enver wasn't interested in the looting. The only thing he was interested in was Chris Woods – who had spoken to Petri in Albanian.

The Australian's satellite phone started to ring.

'Things never cease to amaze me,' he said, close to smiling and never taking his eyes off Enver. 'To think, for instance, that in order for this phone to ring a signal is being sent right now as I speak, out into space and back again. Into space,' he repeated. 'Isn't that amazing?'

★

A florist occupied the ground floor of Sophia's block and the scent of cut flowers hung heavily in the air. David remembered the first time he came here, and how the unexpected scent of flowers had overpowered him into thinking that at midnight the city's Ottoman gardens reappeared, and that it was into these gardens the florist went to gather her flowers.

He called for the lift and waited. Somewhere above, the mechanism started up, but the lift never arrived so he started to walk up the stairs instead.

Following the birth of the Republic and sharp rises in violent crime, the government had set up a Department of Criminology. Sophia, who at the time had been a lawyer for twenty years and was beginning to suffer the same symptoms of nostalgia as others, decided to become a criminologist in order to find out if the emotions of nostalgia she was suffering were true or false. Were crime rates increasing or was it merely that more crimes were being reported? Rape especially. Were they moving forwards or backwards? Had yesterday really been golden or was the golden age yet to come? Was the end in sight?

Sophia and criminologists like her had been trying to fathom the answers to these apocryphal questions for years now, and a certain degree of mysticism had been assigned to this new order of criminologists by other government departments.

Eventually David reached Floor Eleven. The shelves of cacti outside Sophia's apartment, grown to give her mother an occasional excuse for shuffling into the outside world, were still there.

He put his bags down, stretched a hand out to prick his finger on the nearest cactus plant then knocked.

Sophia answered the door in a white blouse and a short black skirt, heavily made up. He had forgotten how tall she was. He felt shabby and suddenly hopeless next to her gaudy glamour.

'Sophia.'

She paused before kissing him, then pulled him through the doorway, taking his bags and carrying them into the corner of the room.

Nothing had changed.

Thick white rugs covered the parquet flooring, so highly polished that it reflected as well as a mirror. The velveteen sofa hugging two of the walls in the room was still on its last legs and the television still a perpetual blaze of light in the corner where

Sophia's mother, a small shrunken woman of eighty-five, was watching *Saturday Night Fever*.

'She's seen it twice this week already,' Sophia said, watching her mother's head nod in time to the music. 'Maybe she's got a crush on John Travolta or something.'

The wall that wasn't taken up with windows or sofa had a large veneer cabinet with glass doors against it. Inside were relics from family holidays in the former Yugoslavia. He had first met Sophia six months after she stopped being Yugoslavian. When, following the saturation of the west's sympathies by the orphans of Ceausescu's Romania, his magazine had decided to slip in some small-scale coverage of the new Republic because somebody on the editorial board had a hunch that their day would come.

'I hope you've eaten. I have to go out.'

This information – meant to be taken lightly – depressed him. 'Where?'

She didn't answer.

'A date?' he said, looking at her clothes again.

She started to move about the room picking up bits and pieces and shoving them into her black leather shoulder-bag.

Her shadow was so tall it stretched across the ceiling as well as the wall.

'Is it love?'

'You know me,' she said. 'It never is. OK. That's everything. You're sleeping in there.' She pointed through the double doors with frosted glass in them.

These led, he knew, to a small sitting room where there was a picture of the Last Supper, painted by Sophia when she had been young enough to have dreams still of becoming an artist. There was more velveteen sofa in there; sofa that would double as his bed.

The apartment felt suddenly more like home than anything he had ever owned in London.

'Mother can put herself to bed.'

David looked over at the elderly woman's nodding head. Apart from this she had shown no signs of life since his arrival.

'She's got John Travolta for company so don't bother trying to talk to her.'

'I'll remember that.'

At the door she paused, her hand gripping the strap of her handbag. 'How many years has it been, David?'

65

'Five.'

She nodded. 'That's right.'

'Why did you ask?'

'I just wanted to make sure you knew.'

'Who's the new man?' he said as she disappeared through the front door.

'A heart surgeon. I'll see you in the morning.'

Despite the warning, he wished Sophia's mother goodnight, but got no response so went into the sitting room, closing the doors as quietly as he could. The shutters in there hadn't been pulled down and he saw himself reflected in the half-light of the room. Beyond his reflected shoulders the whole city lay, and at the edge of it, just before the mountains, was written in neon green across the sky: ALEK. The name of the emperor in its abbreviated form looked to David more like a message. The sort of message a grief-stricken woman would send to the lover she was separated from, through either war or peace, so that he might see it and know she was thinking of him. The four letters suddenly struck him with an overwhelming sense of loss.

Sophia had already made up his bed on the sofa and there was a litre of her home-brewed raki in an old peach juice bottle on the table. Too tired to do anything else – even drink the raki – he sank into the makeshift bed, pulling the blanket round his chin, and wishing that the dialogue from *Saturday Night Fever* was slightly less audible.

Turning over, away from the bottle of raki, he pushed his face into velveteen still covered in dog hairs from Sophia's hound, Luna, now deceased, and fell quickly asleep.

66

17°c

David walked down Ulida Odredi past the hairdresser's and baker's kiosk where he bought a greasy roll with cheese on the top that made him feel sick. At the end, next to the garage, there was a plot of land where two houses used to stand. The plot had recently been purchased by Mr Pulov, the garage owner, who had built sheds on it and filled them with homing pigeons. On the other side of the garage was a courtyard and small corner shop, run by Mr Pulov's Turkish wife.

The man sitting smoking on a stool in the garage forecourt got to his feet with an effort when he saw David. He was wearing a blue boiler suit that had a BP logo across it as well as a couple of splats of fresh pigeon shit on the right-hand shoulder that he seemed unaware of.

'Goran Luković – Sophia's friend.'

He looked David up and down then they shook hands and went into the garage. Inside, green paint was peeling off the walls and there was only space for two cars.

The brand-new, bright red Fiat Punto was parked diagonally across the garage, adopting a car showroom pose.

Goran gave him time to admire it at a distance before going up to the car and gently stroking the bonnet.

David had never been a car man. When on assignment he instinctively strove to blend in, and wasn't entirely sure that the poppy-red Fiat Punto met this requirement.

'You expected something bigger?' Goran said after a while, disappointed. 'I could get you something big – black.' He paused, turning back to the Punto. 'They've got a Cherokee at the pound.'

'A Cherokee?' David edged closer to the Punto.

'Wheels the size of Zastavas.' Goran laughed sluggishly. 'The police've registered it as stolen, but you only need to say the word and they'll have it unclamped and sent over here in no time.'

David wondered what Sophia had told Goran about him. 'A strange way of acquiring rolling stock.'

'Everyone needs to make money.'

David shook his head. 'Forget the Cherokee. This is fine.'

'You like the red? I like the red.'

They stood looking at the car in silence.

'Do I need to fill out any papers or anything?'

'No, you're OK. You paid up front.'

'What if I crash or something?' David asked as Goran got into the driver's seat and manoeuvred the car out of the garage, parking it with precision alongside the kerb.

'You're a friend of Sophia's,' he said, as he got out the car.

David wasn't sure if he was winding up their previous conversation or starting a new one.

'I live the floor above her – Floor Twelve. Maybe we'll see each other.'

David nodded and got into the car.

Goran gestured at him to wind the window down and leant confidentially into the car. 'Bet you think all this is mine, don't you? Garage . . . the lot. Well it isn't – it's Mr Pulov's.'

'I'm sorry.' David couldn't think of anything else to say.

'Free enterprise.'

'It seems to have worked for Mr Pulov,' David found himself stupidly saying.

'You know what *Mr* Pulov used to be? In the old days? He used to be my greaser, that's what he used to be. Son of a bitch,' Goran muttered as he backed away from the car.

As David drove away he saw Goran, through the rear-view mirror, sitting slumped on the stool once more, staring despondently at the pigeons on the other side of the wire fence.

He drove out of the city towards the Aleksandar Palace Hotel where he'd left a message earlier for Guy Spiers, even though the receptionist wasn't interested in confirming whether he was still

68

there or not. David hoped he was. If he wasn't, he somehow felt
that he would be to blame.

He parked in a space reserved for the head chef and got out of
the car. A man wearing a T-shirt that proved he had ridden a
death-defying ride in California at some point in his life came out
of the revolving doors at the front of the hotel, talking to an
American Colonel. He looked familiar – TV familiar.

'The embassy promised me that plane today. I'm meant to be
in Kosovo by 11.00 a.m.'

'Listen, Marvin . . .' David heard the Colonel say.

'Harvey.'

'Harvey. They've got graffiti in Priština . . .' the Colonel mimed
writing on a wall, '. . . President Clinton is King. I've got a jet-
lagged senator who wants to see this. Who wants to see Kosovo
and get his picture taken so he can stick it in a frame on his man-
telpiece back home. The Senator just wants to feel loved. The
crowd cheers, he waves. Even if it only lasts a second . . . he just
wants to feel loved, d'you understand?' The Colonel finished.
'Jesus,' he added, as Harvey Mauser broke down in tears.

At that moment Guy, who had seen David arrive, came
crashing through the revolving doors with wet hair, a red face and
a rucksack on his back. He passed *America Worldwide*'s Harvey
Mauser and the embarrassed Colonel without seeing them.

'I thought you'd forgotten me,' he shouted to David.

'What's that?'

Guy stopped in front of him.

'I thought you'd forgotten me.'

'I had.'

A barely controlled spasm flickered across the young man's face.
Being forgotten was the defining fear of his life.

'But then I remembered you.'

Relieved, Guy clambered into the car.

'I thought you might have upped and left; gone to Thailand –
gone back home. And I figured that if you had gone back home
your girlfriend would soon get tired of your shortcomings as far
as contemporary art was concerned, and cast you adrift. This in
turn might have induced you to – I don't know – run advertising
campaigns for evangelical churches in Brentwood or, worse still,
become an estate agent again.'

Guy didn't say anything.

69

They left the Aleksandar Palace Hotel behind and were soon passing the American embassy.

'What's with the crowds today?' Guy asked.

'I heard that Richard Gere was coming.'

'You're serious?'

David nodded. 'He's flying up to Kosovo for a photo shoot then flying home. A no-expense-spared bit of soul-searching.'

They wound their way back through the city centre, over the river and past the castle.

'Been out the hotel much?' David asked.

Guy, sitting clutching his rucksack, shook his head.

'Have you been out at all?'

Guy shook his head again, and was still clutching his rucksack long after the mosques in the Turkish quarter had disappeared from the rear-view mirror, and they had reached the plains before the mountains where the makeshift tent city came into view.

Violetta walked out of the pharmacist's a hundred yards ahead of Tomo without seeing him. She was still wearing her winter layers and her thin white wrists hung way below the bottom of her coat sleeves.

'Violetta!'

She didn't turn round.

They reached the flower market, which was only just opening up. He followed her into the middle where the smell of Bulgarian roses, at this time of the morning, was overpowering.

Violetta pressed her face against the window of a blue kiosk; a second later the door opened and a woman in overalls appeared. The two women kissed.

'Violetta,' he called out again.

The woman, busy handing her a small spray of flowers, looked over to where he was standing and patted Violetta on the arm.

He watched her remove the headphones her hair had been concealing, and put them round her neck. He could hear, faintly, the bass from the music the machine was still playing.

'Hi,' she said briefly, turning back to the woman so that she could pin the spray to the lapel of her coat.

Tomo turned the other way, watching a man with a trolley full of flower pots trying to negotiate a curb. By the time he turned round again the woman had disappeared back inside the blue kiosk and Violetta had started to walk away.

'Violetta.'

He caught up with her, glancing at the flowers in her button-hole. They were purple and yellow and smelt sweet.

'You were following me?'

'You haven't been at Dal Fufo's.'

They crossed over the road, narrowly missing a bus.

'Is that why you followed me?'

'No.'

For a moment he didn't think she was going to say anything else, but then she did. 'Boris told me you went there to write. I didn't want to interrupt.'

'Boris told you that?'

'He said you wrote short stories. I didn't know you wrote.'

Tomo shrugged. 'It doesn't matter.'

They reached the main crossroads.

'Who else has Boris called in early?'

'Only us.'

They entered the building.

Boris was waiting for them in reception.

'You're here – good,' he shouted, above the noise of the vacuum that the office cleaner was sullenly thrusting backwards and for-wards.

Boris was unusually animated, as if he had at last found the key to something complex he had been labouring over for a long time. Giving the empty water dispenser a friendly thump, he led them into the boardroom, still grey in the early morning light.

Tomo and Violetta sat down at opposite sides of the boardroom table.

Boris went over and stood by the window. He gave a sigh that ended in a pant; something he did when he wasn't sure whether he had gone too far – or not far enough. He started speaking. Words were laborious to him, and this wasn't his usual style. 'You know what happened yesterday? Yesterday wasn't like every other day of my life. Yesterday . . . I had an idea.'

Violetta got a pad and pen out of her bag and put them on the table in front of her.

Tomo stared at Boris, half-afraid that he might be about to take a running jump straight through the plate-glass window like the lawyer on Boulevard Roosevelt three months ago. Although it wasn't yet dangerous to walk the streets through fear of being crushed to death by identifiable flying objects, executive suicide was on the rise.

Violetta drew the dollar sign on her pad, but didn't look up.

'Yesterday, I went to the bar – Dorian's – around nine o'clock. I was feeling low. Not just a bit low, really low.'

'What were you thinking of doing?' Violetta looked up at him. 'Pissing off to Canada? People forget to die in Canada it's so boring, Boris.'

'I thought about Canada,' he admitted. 'I did think about that, but then I met this woman.'

Violetta grunted in disgust.

'No, it wasn't like that. She works for World Refugee Council, that NGO downstairs in the office below us. We got talking about the riot in Stengova camp – did you hear about that?'

'It's hardly insider information,' Violetta responded.

'Yes, but this woman, this . . .' he broke off, got his wallet out of his pocket, and read the card inside, '. . . Angela Fisk, said that they had strong fears of another riot in Stengova camp. The only thing they've been distributing is ready meals – no fresh fruit or vegetables, and no meat. I told her about the warehouse full of our products . . .'

'Did you tell her how long it's been full?' Violetta cut in.

'. . . And she was very interested in the possibility of Republika Foods becoming one of the main suppliers for Stengova camp.'

'Boris, our vegetables come in jars – they're pickled.'

'I know, but at least they're not monochrome.'

Not being partial to expectations, Tomo's blank stare and Violetta's snuffles didn't surprise him. 'Come on,' he goaded them. 'Let me get excited about this. Don't make me do the cynical thing now, Violetta.'

He left the window and walked over to the whiteboard but there were no marker pens.

'In exchange for releasing the goods from the warehouse, she's agreed to think about partial funding for the advertising campaign.'

'What else did you promise her?' Violetta said.

Boris's shoulders quickly sank. 'I said I'd try and get their company's registration speeded up. At the moment they don't even have a bank account, and none of the international staff have had their work visas processed.' He paused. 'Look, neither of you has been paid for the last three months and the bottom line . . . well, we're at the bottom line, and the point is we don't have enough money to run the campaign. We don't even have enough money to refill the fucking Kenco machine and there's hardly going to be an uprising if the supermarkets stop filling their shelves with Republika products. I mean – when was the last time you bought anything produced by this company?'

'Peppers. Two months ago. By mistake,' Violetta said. 'But they're good. You'd never think it from the packaging, but they are.'

'The packaging *is* shit, Boris,' Tomo put in.

'Yeah, it's shit,' Boris agreed. 'I just don't understand choice.'

Nobody said anything.

'I've arranged a meeting with . . .' he searched in his wallet for the card again, '. . . Angela Fisk for this afternoon. I want you both to come with me – give a good impression of the company and maybe find time to talk about the campaign, which is the best one I've seen either of you come up with. Help me to persuade Angela Fisk to spend some of her budget surplus on us?' He broke off. 'What sort of things do you take to a meeting?'

'Business cards,' Tomo suggested.

'Business cards?'

'You know, something with your name, job title, address, contact . . .'

'I know what a fucking business card is, I just don't have any,' Boris said, then suddenly brightened. 'I've got these, though.' He went over to the corner of the room and picked up an old carrier bag, tipping out a pile of cigarette lighters on to the table. 'Can't remember why we had these made – some conference – look, name, address everything. So what do you think about my idea?'

Violetta shrugged.

Boris turned on them.

'All I want you to do is come downstairs with me to the meeting I've organised for this afternoon . . . be polite, maybe even smile, and talk about the fucking campaign.' He stormed out of the room, banging the door back against the wall.

After the initial shock it throbbed on its hinges for a while before swinging gently shut. There was no other sound apart from the distant drone of the vacuum cleaner.

'He's a good man,' Violetta said at last.

'A good man,' Tomo agreed.

They smiled at each other.

John Rudinski was the first to arrive at the meeting scheduled for 11.00 a.m. by the Republic's Bureau for Information and Internal Security. He had been passed along a chain of six different people between reception and the basement room; a pompous procedure that had little to do with necessity and did nothing but put him in a bad mood. Informality for serious meetings was the protocol he was used to.

The riot in Stengova camp had happened and he shared the Ambassador's opinion that there wasn't likely to be another one. The media handled the incident better than anyone had expected and the Ambassador hadn't even considered leaving Priština in order to be here today. No Americans had been injured and no US army personnel would be contributing, now or in the future, to camp security.

Irina Yupović, the President's wife and Bureau's Deputy Head, was sorting through the files in her briefcase and making no attempt at conversation.

Rudinski was trying, unsuccessfully, to match her to the man who had, on that memorable day, taken him pig-shooting. At the memory of this, he instinctively raised his hands to his nose then let them drop again.

'Fuck,' he heard her say under her breath.

She looked up quickly and, seeing that he had heard, said, 'Don't worry, only one of my nails.' She held up her right hand briefly as proof. 'Every time I lose a nail, my manicurist loses a finger.'

The door to the room opened with a bang and Rudinski jumped.

It was the British Ambassador, James Hargreaves, wincing at the noise he'd just made.

He shook hands awkwardly with the President's wife and just as awkwardly with Rudinski. His eyes scanned the table automatically for any snacks or nibbles.

'I had expected to meet on more neutral ground,' Hargreaves said after sitting down, deciding on the spur of the moment that this was a good reason not to apologise for his late arrival.

'Come on,' Irina chastised him lightly, 'not even the moon's neutral any more.'

Rudinski and Hargreaves saw more of each other than either of them wanted to. This was primarily the fault of Hargreaves and his wife for insisting on cultivating their garden themselves. Every time Rudinski stepped out of the house, he was confronted by the sight of the British Ambassador and his wife bobbing up and down on the other side of the hedge – rarely in tandem. Rudinski had seen enough of James Hargreaves – in the garden and at various functions – to realise that he was the sort of man who had lived his entire life during a single definitive week. He had crammed everything he would ever be capable of into that week and was now living in the aftermath.

Last to arrive was Chris Woods, Stengova Camp Manager for World in Crisis, and the man responsible for calling the meeting.

It soon became clear that Dan Hale, the young man with him, had been brought in order to make persistently insensitive and uninformed remarks that only endowed Chris's speeches with an aura of greater wisdom.

Irina Yupović and Chris Woods drove the meeting steadily forward for a full hour, Irina listing the facts of the riot (which she insisted on referring to as an insurrection) with precision. As if she had already discussed the matter with countless others more important than them.

'Anyway, gentleman, maybe riots are to democracies what rallies are to dictatorships – nothing more than showcases.'

With this she suddenly stopped talking and unexpectedly took a back seat.

Rudinski watched her. James Hargreaves watched her. Chris Woods watched her. Despite her immaculate appearance there was something inappropriate about Irina Yupović.

Rudinski couldn't make her out. She wasn't a type, and he needed people to be types. Ellen was a type. Something he had joyed over, and now suffered because of. But suffering was less important than predictability.

'So give them what they want,' Chris Woods wound up. 'And they want Albanian security.' If the meeting had been exclusively Anglo-American, he might have been more droll, but knew that it wouldn't work on the President's wife.

Irina didn't comment or look up from the brief in front of her.

The door to the chamber opened and a young man appeared pushing a tray of coffee and synthetic-looking cakes.

'Albanian security? You mean police?' she said. 'Are you sure that's what you want?'

Chris Woods nodded. 'Camp security has to come first and foremost – we have to do everything we can to ensure that there isn't a re-occurrence of the riot.'

James Hargreaves mumbled in agreement and started to make his way messily through a slice of cake. He only paused once to whisper a warning to Dan Hale that it wasn't real cream, then leant across the table to fill his plate up again.

Rudinski wondered how he managed to keep up the appearance of being malnourished.

'A lot of the refugees in the camp were severely traumatised by their treatment at the hands of Republican police at the border. The riot was inevitable . . .' Chris Woods said, raising his voice.

'The riot was inevitable', the President's wife shouted back, 'because you people have let in far more refugees than the figure the government originally agreed to. As a result of this . . .' with an effort she tried to lower her voice, 'we may have to close the borders again.'

There was silence.

'Get out,' she suddenly yelled.

The two British, American and Australian stared wildly at each other until they realised that she was speaking to the young boy standing motionless with his hands clasped round the trolley bar. He quickly left the room, keeping his head down and dragging the trolley after him.

The next minute a huge extractor fan half-way up the wall started grinding slowly and loudly into life.

This was too much for James Hargreaves, who dropped the piece of cake he was trying to push into his mouth, and watched as the white foam (posing as cream) sizzled and disappeared, leaving a long dark stain along the length of his tie. The remains of the cake fell into his groin and he spent the rest of the meeting surreptitiously trying to pick out every last crumb.

The sound of the extractor fan made the vaulted room feel suddenly more ominous than it had done earlier, and reminded Rudinski of a rumour he had heard about it being soundproof.

'They're arriving by the busload, you can't close the borders,'

76

Chris Woods said heavily, above the persistent clatter of the extractor fan.

'Not me personally, no.'

They all waited but she didn't add anything to this.

'The maltreatment of refugees at the border by Republican policemen is heavily documented . . .' Rudinski put in.

'Were you at the border?' Irina said to Chris Woods, ignoring Rudinski.

He gave no sign either way.

'Because I can tell you now – the day I was there – I wouldn't have wanted a gun in my hand. Imagine being the uniformed minority among sixty thousand terrified, angry people.' She paused.

'Still terrified and still angry,' Chris Woods put in.

'If our police have to go . . . have to be replaced by ethnic Albanian police . . . you wouldn't object to a small base of Republican soldiers being installed just to the north of the village? This is a precautionary measure . . .'

'If you give us ethnic Albanian police, I can assure you that there won't be a need for any precautionary measures.'

'You assure me?'

'Me *personally*.'

James Hargreaves, his hand still in his groin, looked alarmed at the thought of Chris Woods's personal assurance.

'Our methods might be different from yours,' the Australian continued, 'but we're as concerned as you are about possible camp infiltration – of which WIC has intimate worldwide experience. If there are KLA operatives in the camp . . .'

'Of course there are operatives,' Irina said, impatiently. 'Here.' She drew a brown envelope out of her briefcase, shook out some photographs and passed them round the table. 'Photographs of the riot.'

'The Bureau has to be involved,' Rudinski heard her saying to Chris Woods, as he stared at the photograph passed him by Hargreaves. There in the thick of the dust, dismantled fencing and people was his brother-in-law, Peter Miller.

His shoulders tensed. The thought of Peter always overwhelmed him with hopelessness, and the sight of him . . . well. He wondered if anyone here knew. Possibly. He hated the fact that another man's misshapen actions should infringe on his own to such an extent.

'My main concern is the refugees,' Chris Woods said. Then, unexpectedly, 'It really is.'

'Yes.' Irina, who had been watching Rudinski staring at the photo with Peter Miller in it, looked up. 'Yes, I believe it is.'

The red Fiat Punto turned off the main street down a mud lane that followed Stengova camp's newly erected western security fence.

David parked next to two glossy four-wheel drives and with difficulty managed to negotiate the pack of stray dogs that appeared as soon as he got out of the car. This must be the right place. In the Republic, wherever there were stray dogs there were internationals.

David knocked on the door of the house whose address he had been given, but nobody answered.

He guessed that the original occupants had moved out quickly in order to charge premium rates to the new tenants.

Guy walked over to the security fence, nervously hugging his rucksack. He stared through the diamond-shaped wire at the rows of tents with their orderly piles of shoes outside. Some had washing hanging up and there was a constant stream of children passing in and out of the flaps. Men sat smoking in groups.

He watched a young woman washing her hair in a bowl outside one of the tents. She walked to one of the standing taps, her hair white and full of suds, refilled the bowl then walked back to the tent where she began the painstaking job of washing the suds out. He wondered, briefly, whether she was happy or sad at that moment, and guessed that she was probably neither.

David started banging on the door, and after a while it was opened by a short, angry, Italian woman.

'What? What?' she said tucking her shirt into her jeans.

'Is this the office for the organisation Women Against War? I'm looking for Donatella.'

'Somebody's always looking for Donatella. What do you want with her?'

'She's my contact here in Stengova. Her name was given to me.'

'Who by?'

'*Geographica.* The magazine *Geographica.*'

'Oh – you're a journalist.'

David smiled. 'Sort of.'

'Sort of,' she repeated, unconvinced, and finished buckling her belt. 'Is she expecting you? Right now, I mean?'

'She should be.'

A young man appeared in the doorway and squeezed his way past the woman standing there.

'Spatim, wait!' she called out, suddenly distracted. 'Don't go.' She ran down the steps after him, trying to grab hold of his sleeve. Then remembered the audience.

'Got to go, Nadia,' the boy said lightly.

The sun bounced off his Metallica T-shirt. He put his sunspecs on and with a wave to all of them disappeared up the lane.

David turned patiently back to the Italian.

'You'd better come in,' she said, subdued.

David and Guy followed her through the hallway and into a stale-smelling, untidy kitchen. She looked around for a moment, bewildered. A TV set was playing to itself in the corner of the room.

'D'you know when Donatella's likely to be back? Or where I can find her?'

'She'll be in the camp – she's always in the camp. But just you try and find her . . .' She trailed off into a yawn, glanced at Guy then back at David. 'Did you ring beforehand – arrange an exact meeting? You should have rung.'

'I left that to the office.'

She shook her head condescendingly. 'Coffee?'

'Please,' Guy said.

David nodded.

The coffee was belligerently made.

'I work with children in the camp,' she said, and after a few sharp sips of coffee, added, 'I speak Albanian.'

This didn't elicit any response from either of the men.

The next minute they were interrupted by the arrival of a thin, nervous woman whom David guessed immediately to be Donatella.

The energy level in the room changed and Nadia started to buzz around her, speaking rapidly in Italian.

Donatella listened without comment then turned to David. 'Who are you?'

'He's the journalist I was telling you about,' Nadia cut in.

'Are you?' Donatella asked, not willing to take Nadia's word for it.

David smiled apologetically.

Donatella thought about it. '*Geographica?*'

'That's the one. David Everett.' He extended a hand.

'Donatella . . .' She hesitated, about to give her surname. 'Donatella,' she repeated, leaving it at that. Then, worried, 'Women Against War's been badly fucked over by journalists before – I get to see anything you write – proofs – before you go to press. I don't care about deadlines, I have to see the proofs.'

'If I write about you or your organisation, of course.'

'But then,' she said quietly to herself, '*Geographica*'s a magazine so I wouldn't call you a real journalist. I mean', she capitulated, 'working for a magazine like *Geographica*, you're more of a writer, really.'

'Really. Yes.'

She still looked worried. 'So what do you want to see? World suffering?'

'It's the sort of thing I do write about,' David replied.

'"The sort of thing"?' She looked straight at him, into him, as if she had seen all she wanted to see in that split second.

'I thought I would just kind of follow on your tail for as long as you can bear it . . . if I get in the way just kick me to one side.'

Donatella sighed. 'Well, you'd better start following,' she called out, heading towards the front door. 'I've got a meeting in twenty minutes.'

They walked in a line up the lane.

'What's Nadia doing here?' David asked Donatella.

'Didn't she say?'

'She said she was working with children in the camp.'

'She is. Trauma counselling. She's also meant to be co-ordinating a braceleting programme of children under six – to prevent family and child separation during future movements.'

Donatella didn't turn to face him; all he got was her angular profile as she chewed on her nails.

'She was nice,' Guy said, determined that there should be nothing amiss in his brave new world, and definitely no demons. 'Is that the camp?'

Donatella let out a harsh laugh. 'Is he on *Geographica?*'

'No, I met him on the plane. Actually, I brought him along today because he's looking for work.'

For the first time, David became aware that he might be acting irresponsibly.

'For work?' Donatella said to Guy.

'Anything,' he said, but it sounded more helpless than helpful.

'Voluntary?'

Guy hesitated. 'Of course.'

'Have you ever worked with children before? Young people?'

Guy tried to nod and shake his head at the same time. 'I did an arts foundation course in puppetry.'

'Don't worry,' Donatella said, 'you're about as qualified as everybody else in this place. I'll think about it.'

They turned on to the main street, still following the line of security fencing to the right. There was tarmac in places, but it soon gave way to mud again. Every now and then doors in the high walls fronting the main street would open, a woman in a headscarf would poke her head out then pull it back in again. These walls were broken by the façades of a grocery shop, a shop selling electrical appliances, and a pizzeria.

A black BMW with a huge spoiler cruised slowly past and hooted. Spatim, the young man they had seen at the house earlier, leant out grinning.

'That looks high,' David said, pointing to the fence on their right.

'It has more to do with demarcation than security.' Donatella started to chew her nails again. 'Boundaries.'

'So it's got nothing to do with last week's riots then?'

She didn't answer. 'We're going up here.'

They walked under the NATO WELCOME banner then turned left up a street that led (as most streets on the northern side of the village did) to the mosque, which had two minarets – a sign of a community's wealth. They passed the carcass of a cow hanging from a lamppost. The two elderly men sitting beneath it were smoking and laughing, and on a newspaper beside them, the better part of the insides lay sizzling in the noonday sun.

They crossed in front of the mosque and went down another even smaller side street, stopping in front of a building that had been hurriedly purchased by Women Against War even though it was only half-complete.

Looking up, David saw a row of boots swinging above his head that belonged to workmen sitting perched on the edge of the incomplete upper storey. They went inside.

'This is – will be – Stengova's community centre.'

'Must have had a hell of a time getting a project like this off the ground.'

'I did,' Donatella admitted. 'Up until Kosovo, Women Against War has only dealt with the emergency phase of camp planning, but now for the first time we're turning our attention to the post-emergency phase and looking ahead to sustainable development. Only 50 per cent of the refugee population is in camps and collective centres. The rest – at the moment we're estimating around one hundred thousand – are in host families. Some of the households here have taken in up to three refugee families and they don't get compensation for that . . . the least we can do is acknowledge them,' she finished, unable to shake the habit of having to justify her actions to those who funded her visions.

'Right now we're moving forwards with the building because the hodjas are under the impression that the centre's really an annexe to the mosque. The Mayor of Stengova – you should meet the Mayor – thinks that if he backs "in spirit" the building of the centre, we'll cover all the roads in his village with tarmac and ensure that electricity's supplied to all houses.

'Enver Berisha's not a Mayor, he's a baron, and this munici-pality's his fiefdom. You're not taking notes,' Donatella observed.

'I never do – not unless I'm interviewing.'

'This isn't an interview then?'

'No – I'm just keeping my ears and eyes open.'

The beginnings of the community centre were impressive and in one of the downstairs rooms there was already a prayer meeting being held.

'Is the camp population anywhere near stable?'

'Nowhere.'

'I heard that humanitarian evacuation from here and other camps has already started?'

'It has, but on average – across five camps, including Stengova – they're only shifting a thousand a day, and for every one we shift at least another five hundred arrive. They're meant to be setting up a corridor to Albania that should absorb about sixty thousand refugees from the Republic.'

'Involuntary transfer?' David said, watching her.

'We prefer to call it less than fully voluntary transfer. I'm tired,' she broke off, turning to a man who had silently just entered the room. 'Peter! You're late.'

'Got tied up – some professor from the school wanting to put on his production of *Julius Caesar* with kids from the camp. Sorry.'

He looked with interest around the unfinished room.

'This is great.'

'We've got a long way to go.'

'After the hours of Euro pop I've been exposed to with nothing more than a poster of Andie MacDowell to look at and a stack of Oxfam T-shirts, this is great. Believe me.'

'David, this is Peter Miller – our Youth Co-ordinator.'

The two men shook hands.

Nobody introduced Guy.

'So you think WRC would be interested in running youth projects out of the centre?'

'In terms of funding – definitely.'

Donatella opened her second pack of cigarettes that morning. She picked a loose strand of tobacco off her lower lip. 'You know I'll hold you to that, don't you?' she said, flatly, giving her eyes a hard rub.

'You know you won't have to.'

Donatella smiled, pleased for the first time that morning. 'And I've got something for you as well.' She fished behind her for Guy, pulling him forwards by one of his rucksack straps. 'He's looking for work.'

Guy emerged from his stupor and tried to focus.

'He hasn't got any experience, but the good thing about that is, he hasn't picked up any bad habits either. Interested?'

The two internationals weighed the young man up. Peter Miller nodded.

'We haven't got any room left in the WAW house, what about yours?'

'Nothing,' Peter said. 'But I think there's a room going in the MSF house. I'll ask.'

Guy eventually managed to hand over his contact number.

'That looks familiar.'

'It's the number for the Aleksandar Palace Hotel reception.'

'That where you're staying?'

Guy nodded.

'Christ, where do you people come from? It's OK,' he added, seeing Guy's face. 'Don't worry, I'll call you,' he shouted as he left.

Upstairs, supporting pillars had been constructed, but there were no walls and no ceiling. The two-storey building rubbed shoulders with the mosque. The call to prayer at sundown would be deafening.

Impatience passed briefly over Donatella's face when she saw the local builders, sitting with their feet dangling over the edge of the upper floor, but she didn't say anything.

At the back of the upper storey, which was more complete than the front, there was a woman crouched on the floor unloading boxes of books and pamphlets on birth control.

'How's it going, Genevieve?' Donatella said.

'Good, good,' the woman replied, one eye on David who was reading a pamphlet. 'We're open for business.'

Donatella smiled but didn't reply.

'Breed like rabbits here, do they?' Guy said. People had been talking over and through him all morning and he wanted to make some contribution.

The American started to cough. 'Not exactly,' she said, with difficulty. 'It's more an issue of reproductive health; teaching women here the concepts of freedom and choice. I envisage it being a sort of all-round well-woman centre with drop-in mornings, and a crèche. You know.'

Donatella was the only one to nod encouragingly back.

'So the room next door must be for the men's reproductive health programme, then?' David said.

Genevieve gave a tight smile. 'I don't know what the abortion rate among young men here is.'

David and Guy relinquished their pamphlets and they left Genevieve on all fours once more.

'The NGOs can't get enough of reproductive health programmes at the moment. It was the best way of getting funding for the centre,' Donatella said once they were back outside. 'Reproductive health and vulnerable minorities are all the rage at the moment. If we could get some Roma or special-needs kids, the money would come pouring in and we'd have the building finished within the next two months.'

They left the community centre, heading past the mosque and back towards the camp.

Donatella recognised the Mayor's white minibus parked up the side of Petri's and thought about pointing it out to David. But in the end didn't.

On the other side of the street were the two men who had butchered the cow earlier, still sitting on the roadside, still smoking. There was no sign of the carcass or even a drop of blood in the dust around them. The only thing that remained was the beast's head, nestled comfortably at their feet.

Enver parked the minibus where he usually did, down the lane running along the side of Petri's, only this time he had driven round the back way, past the mosque — not up the main village street. The minibus was full of women and luggage. He was tired from the drive and his gut was overwhelmed by the combined smell of sweat and cheap perfume.

At first, when he picked them up at the bus stop on the out-skirts of Sofia — the agreed collection point — they were silent, nervous. Then they all needed to take a pee so he had had to keep stopping the minibus and letting them out. After this, they all started talking to each other at once, and didn't stop jabbering until they hit the border. The guard in Booth 12 at the checkpoint on the Bulgarian border recognised him and waved them through.

Once they crossed over into the Republic, the girls stopped talking again, and none of them had said a word since.

Enver waited for the small group of internationals to pass, then opened the driver's door and got out of the minibus. He recog-nised the Italian woman, but not the two men with her. He walked round to the back of the vehicle and opened the double doors.

Three girls got slowly, warily out.

He shut the door again, signalling to them to follow him through the side entrance and into Petri's.

He was gone about six minutes.

When he got back into the van, he handed the woman sitting up front in the passenger seat a burger wrapped in loo roll. The five women in the back were silent. They smelt the meat. A couple of them watched grease from the burger shining on the woman's chin.

They had been told to pack some food and water, but in Enver's experience they rarely did. Inside Petri's he'd nearly capitulated, and thought about taking burgers out for all the girls in the minibus, but then stopped himself. What the hell was he thinking of? No wonder Emshi never told him anything.

The woman in front finished the burger and tossed the greasy loo roll out of the window.

Enver put the minibus into gear, touching the fabric of Sylvie's skirt.

After months of cajoling, pestering, pleading and bullying he'd finally persuaded her out of the small apartment in Sofia and into a larger one in the Republic's capital that he was renting off a friend. He'd heard from a government contact that they were going to tighten things up on the border and that soon he would need a visa to get in and out of Bulgaria – just like he did for everywhere else. He'd told her that the thought of not being able to get to her when he needed to had driven him mad. He'd told her the truth.

He drove out of Stengova, passing Spatim in his BMW, coming from the opposite direction. They both tooted their horns.

Only one of the women (excluding Sylvie) was staying in the Republic. The other four were passing through en route across Europe and the sea to Essex in England, where they would be met by a car salesman.

This was the only piece of Enver's business that Emshi had nothing to do with. He probably knew about the Bulgarians, but so far, at least, he hadn't interfered.

Enver offered Sylvie a cigarette.

She brushed her hand over his as she took one from the pack. Enver smiled.

When he had pulled up outside the muddy-coloured apartment block in Sofia, Sylvie had let him put her large battered suitcase in the back, and had then automatically climbed into the passenger seat beside him. He liked that.

He tried to keep his eyes on the road, but out of the corner of them he could see her smoking and affecting boredom as she stared placidly out of the window; probably wondering whether her clothes would measure up in the new city. He knew that face. It would give rise to a request disguising itself as a complaint.

He kept his eyes on the road and didn't feel tired any more.

Even though 'mulling' was a new concept to Tomo, he quickly guessed that 'it' would be difficult to execute effectively in a room laid out like a restaurant with large round tables and green leather chairs too heavy to lift. Nobody was sitting down; they were trying to form small groups between tables where a little floor space existed. The windows that nobody had yet successfully reached overlooked the city's main square, still paved with cobbles. You could hardly call it grand. You could hardly imagine that it ever had been grand. Whatever history said about the Ottomans.

The only person he had talked to since Violetta left him standing by the window over an hour ago, was an American in a linen suit, who was desperate to offload some funding a peace-building society had dumped on him, and who had begged Tomo to make a film with it.

'Tomo,' Violetta said, at last reappearing from among the committee-size tables. 'I'd like you to meet Charlie, Cultural Exchange Programmer for the British Council.'

Charlie raised his drink at Tomo. The head of Che Guevara, printed on the front of his T-shirt, was covered in slops from his wine glass.

Tomo stared at Violetta.

The morose, quiet girl had suddenly become fluent and fluid here at the Republic's Writers Club.

'*World in Translation* was Charlie's idea,' Violetta said.

'Yeah, well, I did the same thing in Bosnia,' Charlie agreed loudly. 'Kind of dug around for writers ... found some ... brought them out into the open, and got them translated.' He tried to give a one-handed demonstration of digging for writers, while keeping the glass of wine and cigarette steady with the other. Che's left eye disappeared under a fresh stain. He stopped and looked thoughtful for a moment. '*Writers at War*, that was it. Anthology published by ... well, somebody anyway. Heard of it?' he said, giving Tomo a sideways glance. 'Got rave reviews. People were tripping over themselves.'

Tomo guessed that Charlie was about twenty-eight. Internationals, he had noticed, tended on the whole to look younger than they were.

'Were all the stories about war?'

'Of course. *Writers at War*,' Charlie reminded him. 'Anyway,' he lowered his voice, distracted, 'can't think what else the fucking Bosnians or whatever they are have got to write about.'

'*World in Translation* is a new Balkan anthology,' Violetta prompted him.

Charlie nodded in affirmation. 'They've put me in charge of the whole bloody thing. Now I've just got to find the stuff to put between the covers. Can't tell you how desperate I am — Violetta says you write?' He looked at Tomo, unconvinced.

'You won't get anything out of him now, here,' Violetta said, 'but he can send you some of his short stories.'

'What sort of stuff?' Charlie said, pressing his earlier point. Despite being desperate, he wasn't about to commit himself.

'Please don't give me history, that's all I ask. I've had it up to here with history . . .' He broke off to signal to a girl walking around the room with two bottles of wine. Up close, she smelt badly of stale sweat, not helped by the fact that her white blouse was 100 per cent polyester. Charlie wrinkled his nose as she filled his glass, sniffing the wine suspiciously afterwards. 'Might as well,' he said, raising his glass. 'After all — British Council's paying. Yeah, well, just no more history. If I have to read one more fucking short story about Night of the Long Knives or any of that stuff, I mean it's just so . . . used. Not even just used,' he said, warming to this, 'but overused, you know. I'm telling you,' he whispered, 'I've had it with Europe. Once this Kosovo stuff blows over I'm out of here. Tel Aviv — now that would be somewhere.'

He gulped the glass of wine down and looked around for the bad-smelling waitress.

Outside, the night was warm.

Tomo and Violetta crossed the square towards the old bridge over the Vardar, leading to Casa Baba, the Turkish quarter. There weren't many people around.

'What was all that about?'

'What about?'

'You in there.'

She was back to her usual shrunken self. There was no sign of the technicolour she had been displaying all evening.

'I don't know how you persuaded me to come tonight,' he mumbled.

'Haven't you been to the Writers Club before?'

'Course not.'

As they reached the bridge and started to cross it, Tomo narrowly missed a cardboard box whose occupant was a one-month-old baby about the length of his foot, lying on its back in a striped jumper.

88

'You haven't even read any of my stories,' Tomo added.

'Look, Charlie's hardly going to put a great deal of effort into looking for his "stuff" – he'll just publish any crap to hand.'

'Thanks.'

'But that's just the point – you're not crap.'

'How do you know?'

'I just know.' She was walking fast, not looking at the river on either side of them or the other small cardboard boxes dotted around the bridge. 'Can I read your stories?'

He didn't answer. 'How do you know Charlie?'

'I know a lot of British Council people.'

They stopped in the middle of the bridge.

Violetta at last turned to face the river.

'That day in Dal Fufo's when I said you went to the same school as me and you never answered . . . you did. Afterwards, I remembered. You were the girl they sent to Berlin to study on some programme for exceptionally gifted children,' he said, turning to her.

'Mathematics – I was sent to study mathematics.'

'It was you. The papers were full of it: Violetta Nebkov. Child genius.'

'The problem is, I came back. You're not meant to come back from places like Berlin. It isn't easy to put hope into a person, and even less easy to forgive them if they don't fulfil that hope.'

She broke away from the parapet she had been leaning against and carried on walking.

'As a nation we have an overwhelming desire to turn ordinary men and women into heroes – have you noticed that? I don't know whether it's Communism or whether we've always had an insatiable appetite for heroes; even now – that's why we make such depressing democrats. So-called freedom makes poor soil for heroes to grow in.'

'I don't believe in heroes,' Tomo said. 'They're completely at the mercy of history.'

'Maybe,' Violetta agreed. 'But we're still good at heroes – here in the Republic.'

They reached the other side of the bridge where there were a couple of Roma women standing talking. Tomo wondered which one of them was mother of the baby in the striped jumper, lying in its box on the other end of the bridge.

'Why did you leave Berlin?' he asked, as they walked up a flight of wide low-strung steps with a mosque on either side.

'That's exactly what my mother asked when I phoned from the bus station.'

'What did you say to her?'

'In Berlin, I discovered that no matter how much numbers are used to corrupt, they themselves remain incorruptible . . . they're ideal. Think about it – numbers are the only unfallen things in existence that we're able to touch.'

'You said that?'

'No, I told her I got homesick.'

They passed an office building on their left with a brand-new motor scooter parked outside. This was the Republic's Lotto HQ, and that week's lucky numbers flashed over Tomo and Violetta as they crossed the forecourt.

'That was the last time I spoke to her.' Violetta paused. 'I really did get homesick.'

The streets got narrower and busier. Most of the shops in this quarter were still open.

'Who buys those?' Tomo said, pointing to a string of traditional shoes, in all sizes, strung round a shop doorway.

'I don't know – tourists?'

'There aren't any tourists.'

Violetta shrugged. 'Are you hungry?'

Tomo shook his head. 'Tired.'

'I go there most nights to eat.' She pointed out a long building with small windows. 'It's a kind of cafeteria for factory workers. The food's good, and in winter – because they cook on an open fire – it's like a hothouse. My apartment doesn't have heating so that's where I go.'

'I'll see you home,' he offered.

'This is home.'

She opened a door at the side of the jeweller's shop they were standing in front of.

Tomo saw a long shabby hallway with blue tiles – some of them smashed – and the dim outline of a table at the end.

'In there?' he said, not quite believing her.

She said, 'You'll get some stories to me? For Charlie?'

Tomo laughed a short cynical laugh.

'Don't hate him – you don't need to. He's lonely, that's all. You should never underestimate the lengths people go to for warmth and company.'

There it was again, that something he'd often felt in her presence that made him hold his breath.

'Is that what it is with you and Boris?' Tomo said, suddenly articulating something that had been lying half-formed at the back of his mind all day – ever since that morning's meeting.

She stepped into the hallway of her apartment and for a minute he thought she was going to shut the door in his face. But she didn't.

'Can I tell you something?'

Tomo waited.

'I loved my parents. I had absolute faith and trust in them – I mean, I loved them unconditionally. When I got back from Berlin I found out that their love for me was only conditional. That's the sort of discovery no child should have to make – especially one who's managed to think otherwise – through sheer perseverance and need – for seventeen years. The shame of my return from Berlin was too much for them. I had nowhere to go. That woman in the blue kiosk at the flower market this morning, she found me. She lives in an apartment in the western side of the city that she shares with her brother . . .'

'Boris,' Tomo finished.

'Boris,' Violetta repeated. 'She called him that day and he came to the flower market to pick me up. He called me kid – nobody's ever done that. I started a job tying bouquets at the flower market, saved some money and he helped me get this apartment.'

She was playing with the door, pushing it gently backwards and forwards with her hand, staring at his feet on the pavement outside.

'That's more than I ever intended telling anybody. You should go home now.'

'Have you seen your parents since?'

She carried on staring at his feet. 'You should stop caring about the things that don't matter and start caring about the things that do. Firstly because there are less of them, and secondly because if you don't start soon, you'll never change anything.'

'You think I can?'

'You should go now.'

Without another word, she did close the door this time, gently but firmly in his face.

He stared at the shut door, waiting for it to open, but it didn't, and no sounds came from behind it either.

He made his way across the street to the workers' cafeteria she'd pointed out earlier to him, and went inside.

Irina Yupović was sitting on the bed, her briefcase beside her. When the President poked his head round the door, she held up her hand for five more minutes, then went back to reading the papers in front of her.

Despite the President having a country to run twenty-four hours a day, this small gesture of his wife's made him feel suddenly useless. He sighed and poured himself a vodka.

Irina had trained, like many women of her generation, as an engineer, but when the opportunity arose decided, instead, to accept a position at the Bureau for Information and Internal Security.

When they first met, decades ago, she had warned him that she wasn't very good at resisting temptation, which had proved true. This coupled strangely with her other affliction of always telling the truth.

He sat down on a chair where he had a clear view of her through the open bedroom door. Through the wall he could hear faint strains of music coming from Elena's room that he had asked her to turn off over an hour ago.

His wife put her papers away, clicking the briefcase shut.

'The Australian today – the one running Stengova camp – he knows that the riot was started by KLA operatives who are still in the camp. And if they're still in Stengova then so are the arms,' she said abruptly, then sighed.

'I asked her to turn that bloody thing off over an hour ago – she still hasn't done it,' the President said, suddenly annoyed by the constant beat making its way through the wall. 'He knows about the arms?'

'Definitely. I'd say through a combination of suspicion, experience and intuition.'

'Did you talk about all of this in front of the British Ambassador and that American Jew?'

'Of course not. We invited them in order not to talk about it in front of them.'

'What's the Bureau going to do?'

'What they want – withdraw the Republican police force and have them replaced by Albanian security.'

'Do we have any Albanian police?' the President asked.

'Only 3 per cent.'

He turned to look fully at her. 'This Australian – he's playing with you.'

'Only because I let him.'

'But you must believe him at least half-capable of uncovering the arms,' he said, continuing to observe her.

'He's got a three-week window. If he doesn't flush out the operatives by then, we'll be installing a small base of Republican soldiers just to the north of the village in the foothills.' She hesitated. 'But I think he will.'

'You do?'

The telephone started to ring.

He answered it. It was the American Ambassador.

'Mr President?' the voice on the other end of the line said, surprised at the simplicity of dialling a number and, after a few rings, being able to speak directly to the President of the Republic.

The President let out a wary, 'Yes?'

'Mr President?' the Ambassador said again, to convince himself.

'Speaking.'

'Of course, of course.' Pause. 'It's come to my attention that the Serbian Ambassador, whose private residence is, as you know, opposite our own, has mounted a small exhibition of photographs along the railings outside the front of his residence.

'You will understand, sir, I'm sure, how offensive not only myself but the American government finds this impromptu exhibition.'

'Exhibition?' the President said, bewildered.

'Yes. Exhibition of photographs.'

'But photographs of what?'

'Belgrade,' the Ambassador said heavily.

The President, quick to see his own point but often slow to see that of others, couldn't fathom the American's outrage.

'You know. Belgrade,' the Ambassador said with even more weight this time.

The President frantically tried to remember if Belgrade was in fact not Belgrade at all, but code for something else.

'There are photographs mounted outside the Serbian

Ambassador's residence depicting bomb damage in Belgrade. Material and human. The headlights of my car illuminated this photographic exhibition when we returned home from a function fifteen minutes ago.'

'Ah, the bombing,' the President said, relieved at last to get to the bottom of the matter.

'There are pictures of human victims,' the American stressed, 'and I can assure you that they aren't a pretty sight.'

'But the pictures are true?'

'Of course they're true. What are you talking about?' the other man said, giving in to his irritation. 'It's what happens when something gets bombed.'

'A city. When a city gets bombed.'

'Me and my family have to pass these pictures every day,' the Ambassador said. Then paused. 'I expect your full co-operation on this.'

The President was nodding, temporarily forgetting that they were holding the conversation over the telephone and that the Ambassador needed to hear and not see his consent.

His wife lay down on the bed, her face turned towards him.

'For Christ's sake, I have children,' the American shouted.

The President must have misheard him because he replied, raising his voice for the first time, 'We're all children.'

21 °c

David headed to one of the city's largest shopping malls. The meeting at the American embassy wasn't until 10.30 a.m. and, feeling guilty that he had been too drunk to buy Sophia any perfume from duty free on the way over, he now bought her two bottles of the only recognisable type he could find – something that brought the wrong kind of smile to the pharmacist's face.

After this he went into one of the marginally less depressing internet cafés that occupied at least one in every five shop units. He had a coffee, sent an e-mail to Sally at the *Geographica* offices in Washington, failed to think of anyone else who might be expecting an e-mail from him, then left.

It was still just 10.00. The only thing he could think of doing to kill time was walking up the hill the castle stood on.

He hadn't expected to see anybody, but when he reached the top there were already three other people up there – a couple of female K-For soldiers giving an American Colonel a flirtatious morning tour of the ruins.

At one time he would have been able to imagine the castle in its entirety . . . the people who used to live there . . . right down to the finest costume detail. Now all he could see were ruins, and in front of them the wide glacial Vardar cutting through the centre of the city. Beyond the river were the mountains – some of the tops still covered in snow – and beyond the circle of mountains

95

the things he couldn't see, but that he knew were there . . . moving clockwise . . . Albania, Serbia, Kosovo, Bulgaria . . . Greece. So many frontiers, and not an ocean in sight. He felt suddenly an islander's panic and exhilaration. I don't have to stay here, I can go anywhere, he thought. The sound of freedom for a brief moment, deafening.

He made his way towards the castle's only remaining portcullis. On a parapet just to the side of this a local rock group was standing, dressed in black and silver, having some publicity shots taken. There was no sign of the K-For soldiers or the American Colonel. Passing under the portcullis, he walked back down the hill and on to Boulevard Partisanska.

It took a while to get through passport control at the American embassy gates because the two large security guards on duty had no record of his appointment. In the end they reluctantly buzzed him through.

Once inside, the embassy felt clean, new and bullet-proof; more of a compound than an oasis. He waited in reception for ten minutes before a young woman who was neither attractive or un-attractive, just clean, new and bullet-proof like everything else, took him upstairs to the Vice-Ambassador's office in the visa department.

They made their way through a maze of screens and pot plants that looked plastic despite being real, until they came to a halt outside an office door. The girl knocked and pushed him gently inside.

'Tea? Coffee?'

'Coffee, please.'

'Sure. No problem.'

She was gone.

The man facing him was younger than he had expected, but David guessed he had more years' experience than his face gave him credit for.

'Rudinski – John,' he said pleasantly. 'I'm a subscriber to *Geographica* – very pleased to assist.' He stretched and looked out of the window. 'I saw you cross the road.'

'You did?'

This observation unsettled David.

The girl pushed a cup of coffee silently round the door and he tried to drink it without slurping, feeling instinctively that slurps would annoy Rudinski.

96

'Quite a time to start your term of office,' David said.

Rudinski eased himself further into his chair.

'What with the war and everything.'

Rudinski shrugged and said, 'I was in Albania when it blew.'

This bravado, which reared its head only occasionally, was as close to sporting moments as Rudinski liked to come.

'And it certainly blew,' David added warmly.

'It did, didn't it,' Rudinski said, laughing suddenly.

Without knowing why, David started laughing as well.

The girl poked her head round the door.

'Everything OK in here?' she said, as if she had given them extra playtime – unsupervised.

'Everything's fine,' Rudinski responded.

Once she'd closed the door, he sat up straight again.

'You want to know about visas, right?'

David nodded.

'Well, I'll tell you what I can – sorry you can't speak to the Consul.' The way Rudinski said this made the Consul seem like his senior and not his junior.

'In light of the . . . the conflict . . . visa applications have of course increased. You saw the queue stretching along the front of the embassy when you came in? That's there from sunrise to after sundown. Most of them are Albanian and have just driven across the border – jumping on the bandwagon – not Kosovar Albanian.' His tone suggested that this opportunism wasn't something, on a personal level, he necessarily disapproved of. 'They think we don't know the difference.' He allowed himself a low laugh. 'Most of the cars in that parking lot opposite are stolen Mercedes with Tirana plates on.'

David had already noted this, before entering the embassy, but he didn't want to spoil the Vice-Ambassador's enlightenment session, guessing that he was someone who clammed up easily.

'And the stories they tell. Stories as tall as . . . as tall as,' Rudinski tailed off, shaking his head, then got up and went over to the window, looking for something as tall as the stories he'd heard.

'We had this guy in here once, claiming that a donkey dropped out of the sky and crippled him. He needed to go to the US for urgent medical treatment. He wasn't even Albanian . . . Montenegrin or something.' Rudinski turned to face him. Smiling, but preoccupied. 'A diplomat's anecdotes.'

97

'I think they're more than that,' David said.

Rudinski looked interested.

'I've often found that, in the line of duty, many diplomats end up getting more of a soul than they've bargained for.'

Rudinski moved nervously away from the window and sat down. 'Anything else you'd like to ask?' he said, in his pleasant tone again.

'How did Richard Gere's state visit go?'

'Fine. Just fine.' He turned round a small photo-frame on his desk and David saw the Vice-Ambassador with his arm slung round the actor's shoulders.

'And can you tell me if it's true that Hillary Clinton's coming to the Republic next week?'

'Well now, there's a lot of people coming here. It's the place to be, you know,' Rudinski said, turning the photograph back round to face him.

David was irritated – he thought Rudinski might have given him this.

The phone on the desk started to ring.

David stood up but Rudinski signalled at him to stay with one hand while picking up the phone with the other.

'Hello? She's what? What d'you mean they won't let her through? She's my wife.' He slammed the receiver down and yanked open his office door.

His secretary put her phone down and they continued the conversation face to face.

'Has she not got her passport? Is that it? I'll phone down.'

'The passport's not the problem,' the secretary said with a sigh. 'It's the fact that she's got a dog with her.'

'A dog? But we don't have a dog.'

The secretary didn't say anything.

Rudinski stood there staring straight through her.

'So what d'you want me to say? I've got them on hold,' she said.

'Who?'

'Security.'

'Tell them I'll be right down.'

The secretary took the phone off hold. 'He'll be right down.' She spun round in her chair and went back to work.

David noticed that she said 'he' and not 'Mr Rudinski' when speaking to security.

'We might have to call it a day,' Rudinski said, standing up.

David put his notepad away and followed the Vice-Ambassador downstairs, back through the maze of screens and pot plants. They crossed the immaculate reception and went into security where three guards stood close to Ellen Rudinski, who was holding a wounded dog in her arms.

'Mr Rudinski, please,' the tallest guard said, stepping forward, as if they'd been locked in unreasonable argument for hours.

Rudinski ignored him. 'Ellen?'

'John, I think it's broken its leg.'

'Ellen.' Rudinski sounded suddenly exhausted.

'I'm sorry, Mr Rudinski, but we couldn't let your wife in with the . . .'

'Shut up. Please. Will you just shut up.'

The guard stood with his fists on his hips. He would remember this.

'Did you run into the dog, Ellen? Is that it?'

She shook her head.

'With the car?' He looked impatiently round the room. 'Could you leave us alone for a minute?'

The guard with the fists still on his hips shook his head.

'Sorry, Mr Rudinski,' one of the others added.

'I wasn't in the car. I was walking.'

'You walked from the house?'

'I wanted to see some animals. I thought it might help.'

'You went to the zoo?'

'I was going to the zoo but then I found this dog by the side of the road.'

Her husband stared at her.

She waited patiently, then sighing said, 'So d'you think it's got a broken leg?'

The guards started talking among themselves.

Rudinski took in the blood on the front of his wife's trousers. There was a smudge on her face, and her hands and arms looked sticky with it. Last of all he looked at the dog.

'The dog's dead,' he said. 'The fucking dog's not even alive.'

'That's not true,' Ellen blurted out, her eyes shining with tears.

'Give me the dog.'

She backed away.

He looked down at his security pass that had got tangled in his tie.

'You're tired, Ellen.'

'I'm never tired.'

'Why don't you put the dog down and we'll take you home.'

She stared sullenly at him.

David stood watching this exchange between husband and wife. He heard Rudinski's tired voice and the talk of the security guards behind him, which sounded smutty even though it wasn't.

For a moment he met Ellen Rudinski's eyes, and he looked away before she did.

'I'll take Mrs Rudinski home,' he heard himself suddenly saying.

The Vice-Ambassador turned to stare at him. He'd clearly forgotten all about him.

'You've got a car outside?'

'No, but I can get a taxi.'

'A taxi?' John Rudinski bowed his head and moved it slowly from side to side, a helpless smile on his face. 'I could get an embassy driver take her home.'

'A taxi would be better. The Aleksandar Palace is just up the boulevard. You've got taxis pounding down Partisanska by the minute.' David paused. 'Have you never noticed that?'

Rudinski looked at him. He was talking about the real world where there were taxis and hotels.

Nobody said anything.

'D'you want to leave the dog here and go home now?' David said at last.

Ellen carried on looking at him, only she wasn't looking so much as watching.

'He must be heavy for you,' David tried.

'How d'you know it's a "he"?'

David shrugged. 'You just do. With dogs.'

She gave a quick laugh, which only seemed to make her husband more tense.

To David, she said, 'I think you're right.'

With a preoccupied smile, she laid the dog down on the conveyor belt running under the X-ray machine.

He felt sorry for the security guard, who would have to clear up the mess.

Ellen Rudinski stood waiting by the door, expectant now.

John Rudinski looked out of the window, past his wife standing in security in bloodstained clothes, at the queue stretching along the road.

'I can't thank you enough,' he said at last, turning to David. 'Really I can't.'

Ellen was smiling her amused smile, as if she'd caught him out. He tried hard not to look at her.

'But maybe I should take her home myself?'

David waited patiently for him to work it out.

The security guards started moving over towards the X-ray machine and the dog.

'No. I think I'll take you up on your offer if you don't mind. Wait – my card – it's got our address on it.'

'I know our address,' Ellen said.

'Will you take the card?' He handed it to David. 'I've got your details.'

David was handed his passport back by one of the guards then left the embassy, followed by Ellen Rudinski.

Husband and wife parted without exchanging another word.

For a moment Rudinski wondered what on earth he'd done. Instinct told him he was getting enmeshed, but in what exactly, he had no idea. The only thing he did know for sure – and it was the first thought he had had – was that he would never have found Irina Yupović standing in security at the American embassy with a dead dog in her arms.

'Christ, it's hot.'

Dan Hale walked into the UNHCR field office in Stengova, got himself an iced water from the machine, and flopped. He stared at his colleague, Olive, then stared out the window at his 4x4, parked outside.

It hadn't rained for weeks, which irritated him. Back in February the potholes in the road had been full of rainwater and he had derived inordinate amounts of pleasure from driving through them at high speed, spraying up tunnels of water.

He was about to try and make conversation with Olive when the door opened and Guy Spiers from Youth Services walked in.

'Looking for someone?' Dan said.

'Suma . . . Suma.'

'The big fat Paki?' Dan asked pleasantly.

Olive looked up. 'Dan,' she said, pro forma.

'Sorry, the gentleman of Asian descent.'

He felt Olive's eyes on him as she pushed her long, straight, greasy hair off her greasy face and behind her greasy ears. She was only here because her boyfriend – a Barclay's Bank Manager in Reading – hadn't proposed to her. She might not like Dan, but she still expected him to make a pass. Something he hadn't yet been desperate enough to do.

She gave him a final squint before bending her head over the volume of Excel printouts once more.

'He was meant to be getting hold of some loudspeakers for us. For the youth tent.'

'I heard him say something about that,' Olive said, looking up again, her pen in her mouth.

Guy looked round the office.

'I don't see any speakers.'

'That's the problem with Suma,' Dan said. 'Unreliable.'

'We've got tents arriving from the warehouse this afternoon and you've also got a meeting with Gary some time later. Don't forget that,' Olive reminded Dan.

'Who's Gary?'

'The permaculture man.'

'The one who grows vegetables – wants to turn the camp into an experiment in organic farming? I've never had a meeting with him later than 11.00 a.m. Any time after that, he's pissed.'

Guy got to his feet.

'Where're you going?' Dan asked, bored.

'I'll catch up with Suma later.'

'What do you want with loudspeakers anyway . . . planning a party?' Dan called out.

But Guy had already left the offices and disappeared behind the 4x4.

There was even more dust in the camp than usual, Guy noted as he walked through the northern section and down the field towards the southern. Then he saw the reason why. There was a large flat-back lorry pulling up by the youth tent.

He watched as a red-faced man with a beard got out and stared around him.

By the time he reached the lorry, Peter Miller had emerged from the tent.

The lorry driver said something, smiling.

'What's he saying?'

'It's not Albanian,' Peter said.

The strains of Alba pop could be heard coming from inside the tent.

'Or French,' Guy added.

'You speak French?'

He nodded.

The lorry driver, now making expansive gestures with his hands, led them round the back of the truck to where hundreds of metres of rope lay coiled among folds of red and yellow oil-cloth piled as high as the driver's cab and tied on badly with fraying blue string.

'It's a circus tent,' Guy said, suddenly.

Peter nodded slowly, ready to believe this. 'A donation maybe.'

Half an hour later, the red-and-yellow striped circus tent was lying in a heap at the side of the truck, a crowd standing around it.

'What are all these people doing here?' Guy said to Nadia, who had just emerged from another tent close by where she was helping with the under-fives' rehearsal of *Little Red Riding Hood*.

'They think it's the UNHCR tents arriving,' she said, looking at their faces.

The driver was still talking in his unidentifiable language.

'Well, it's not Italian,' Nadia said.

'Nobody knows what it is.'

'I don't know what to do with him, his lorry or his tent,' Peter said.

Guy stood back and felt his elbow knock into somebody. He turned round. There was a girl standing behind him with her hand over her jaw.

'Really sorry – you OK?'

She took her hand away and he recognised the girl he had seen washing her hair the first day he arrived in Stengova. He was sure it was her.

'Nadia,' he said, pulling at the Italian's arm. 'Tell her I'm sorry.'

'Who? What did you do?'

She turned round and saw Aida standing there. She hadn't spoken to her since the last time she'd tried to get her to come to one of her trauma-counselling sessions.

'Tell her I'm sorry. About her jaw,' Guy urged.

Nadia turned and said something in Albanian to Aida, who moved away.

'Where's she gone?'

'She was waiting for the tents – she thought this was the UNHCR delivery like everyone else. Not some circus tent from God knows where.'

'She's sleeping out?'

'Thousands are – tarpaulin.'

'I know about the tarpaulin,' Guy said, irritated.

He hung around for a few minutes more then started to walk slowly away, back towards the UNHCR field offices.

Ellen Rudinski either hadn't noticed or didn't care about the blood on her clothes. David could see her through the rear-view mirror, staring out the window. The radio was on and he sat listening as the DJ kept getting interrupted by ads for new furniture stores and sports shops.

The driver took the long way round and when they stopped, half-way up the hills in the middle of the diplomatic district, gave the meter a thump to send the fare up. Even though he was paying, David let all this pass.

The driver's face was expressionless, uninterested.

David got out the car, but Ellen Rudinski showed no sign of moving.

He walked round to her side, opened the door and helped her out.

They stood by the open gates at the top of the drive as the taxi pulled away, listening to it screech its way back down the hill.

David looked at the card the Vice-Ambassador had given him, checked the address and started to walk up the drive, followed silently by Ellen Rudinski.

Over the hedge in the house next door, a woman in a peach kimono opened her front door, which seemed miles away, looked out towards the road, saw David and Ellen then quickly shut the door again.

Out the corner of his eye, David saw Ellen glance at her neighbour's closed front door.

They reached the porch. There were logs piled inside it. He couldn't imagine John Rudinski chopping logs.

David looked up at the house then back at the garden whose length they had just walked. He didn't realise they had houses this big in the city.

'Keys?' he said to Ellen.

She stared blankly at him.

'Keys to the house?' More impatiently this time.

Another taxi pulled up in the road. A young man with black hair and a black goatee, wearing a suit, got out empty-handed.

The front door of the neighbouring house opened again and there was the woman in the peach kimono standing with her arms wrapped around her.

This time she didn't look over the hedge. She didn't take her eyes off the young man walking down her drive.

The man went inside and the door closed.

'I don't have keys,' Ellen Rudinski said, more to herself than David. 'I mean, the door's open.'

David gave it a push and they went inside.

Ellen put her hand to her head.

For the first time he wondered how on earth he was going to get back to the city centre and cursed himself for not asking the taxi to wait.

'You OK now?' he said.

Ellen looked up, at last acknowledging him. 'Now?' She smiled.

He watched her slowly trying to pull herself together, but her mind was elsewhere.

'I think I'll go and change.'

She went upstairs, leaving him in the hallway. He didn't know whether to stay or go; he didn't know whether he wanted to stay or go.

Five minutes later she walked back down the stairs slowly, as if trying to steady herself – cleaned up and looking twenty years older. She'd sort of done her hair, and sort of done her make-up and he felt more sorry for her than he had done when she'd stood in embassy security with the dead dog in her arms.

She wasn't surprised to see him still standing there and that annoyed him.

'You want a drink?'

She showed him into the breakfast room at the back of the house then disappeared into the kitchen.

Indoors, the vestiges of a former charm still hung around her, and he guessed that she was the sort of woman who used to have a way with men.

He heard the glass doors of a cabinet opening and an ice-tray being pulled out of the freezer. A few seconds later the ice was dropped into glasses and had something poured over it that made it crack.

'What a view,' David said, staring out over the city.

'Yeah.' She came back into the room with two glasses in her hands, but didn't look out of the window. 'I'm sick of views. Thank you . . .' she added, handing him his drink, '. . . for bringing me home. You handled me well. That's what I was thinking when I was upstairs changing.' She paused. 'And I'm not even your type, am I?' She gave a painful cracked smile. The effort of trying to drag up the old charm.

'No, you're not.'

She liked this. 'We don't have to flirt then.'

They were both standing by the window now, neither of them looking at the view.

'I know your type,' she said.

'You do?'

She nodded, but kept it to herself for a while. 'The unbreakable sort. That's your type.'

He didn't say anything.

'Jesus, I break in half just getting out of bed in the morning.'

She took a sip of her drink and sighed with relief.

David recognised the sigh.

'Your daughters?' He pointed to the two photographs in the bookshelves. He was surprised – he hadn't pictured the Rudinskis with offspring.

'Uh-huh.' She didn't ask him if he had any children. 'You want to go out into the garden?'

She slid the patio doors back.

'All the home comforts here,' she said, indicating the built-in barbecue to the left-hand side. 'You should have seen Albania.'

'I have seen Albania.'

David wanted to finish his drink and leave, and guessed she probably wanted to do the same, only she couldn't leave because this was her house and she had nowhere else to go.

She sat on the sun lounger, and he sat at the table unable to find a comfortable position.

They sat in silence.

After a while they heard a series of low cries, gradually but unevenly increasing in pitch and volume.

They turned, instinctively, towards the house next door – listening to the woman in the peach kimono reach her climax – and still couldn't think of anything to say. They waited, sitting it out until the man let out two yells.

Ellen Rudinski closed her eyes, and David thought she was asleep until she said, 'That was Anne Hargreaves.'

He nodded, as if the name was familiar.

'The British Ambassador's wife.'

She opened her eyes, turned her head sideways to stare at him, then shut her eyes again. 'I like Anne Hargreaves.'

'I should go.'

'You don't want another drink?'

'I do want another drink, but I should go.'

He stood up, ready to walk back through the house and let himself out, but she somehow managed to get to her feet.

'I need to write,' he said, suddenly angry that she hadn't asked him his name yet.

'You're a journalist? I thought you were a journalist.'

She was lying, saying anything that came into her head now. She still didn't ask him his name.

They reached the front door.

'Wait.' She picked up her handbag from the chair in the hallway. 'My card. I should give you my card.'

'Your card?'

'All Ambassadors' and Vice-Ambassadors' wives get them. Don't ask me why.'

He watched as she fumbled with her wallet.

'Who's that?' he said, looking at the snapshot slotted sideways into the wallet.

'My brother.'

'What's his name?'

'Peter. Peter Miller.'

'Peter? The name's not familiar, but the face is . . . wait, Stengova – that's where I've seen him. At the camp.'

'You've been to Stengova?'

'That's where he works?'

She nodded, not sure if David knowing Peter was a good thing or not. She felt it meant something, but wasn't quite sure what and wished she hadn't got out of the habit of thinking straight.

'World Refugee Council, that's who he works for. You're in touch?'

'Always.'

She opened the door, looking blank again.

'I'm sorry about the dog,' he said.

'The what?'

'The dog.'

He waited for her to remember, but she didn't say anything else.

'Hello – see you around – yeah, well – lay me five – shit.'

Aida went over her English lexicon in her mind while watching the man in the purple trousers, whom she didn't like, talking to her father. The one who gave her loose smiles and made her father feel important. The Albanian who had been to America.

She knew he was watching her as well. Watching her smoke the cigarettes he'd given her two days ago, that she'd held off smoking until now. Just her luck that at the moment she finally lit up, he appeared. She smoked slowly and sullenly, knowing that if she looked up and caught his eye he'd try and smile.

Benny Schmalz shook her father's hands with both of his, then walked off without trying to speak to her.

Aida watched her father's uneven but triumphant approach back to the tarpaulin. He was proud to be seen talking to a man like Schmalz.

She took hold of him under the elbows and eased him into a sitting position as he mumbled something into his moustache.

'That man thinks,' he said with a slight groan as he folded his legs under him. 'He thinks.'

He gave her a brief almost guilty glance out of the corner of his eye.

She finished her cigarette but didn't ask him what he had been talking about, although she knew he wanted her to.

Silence had been her mother's tactic, born of pride and resulting in violence. Aida didn't have tactics and she didn't play games; she had plans.

The man she called father had spent his entire life knowing that his wife would never have married him of her own free will. Her pride overwhelmed him and he was forever trying to break her up into something more digestible.

Aida was constantly surprised by the fact that he had never killed her mother.

Once she had walked into a room late at night to find her mother sitting on her father's lap. He was crying and trying to talk to her and she was sitting there motionless.

She remembered this occasion vividly, but was still trying to work out if it was of any use to her or not.

Confident that Benny Schmalz was out of sight, she was about to light a second cigarette when she saw Guy Spiers walking towards them, carrying something heavy in his arms.

She knew – instinctively – that he was going to stop at their tarpaulin; and that the heavy object he was carrying was a tent.

He stopped about a hundred yards away, put the tent down and paused for breath. When he picked it up again he started to walk more slowly, as if he thought a rapid approach would make them afraid. He stopped again, by the tarpaulin this time.

Aida stared at his boots, which were brown and covered in dust.

Her father had worked the whole thing out as well, but wouldn't look at the man.

'Why's he giving us the tent?' he asked, giving her the same guilty sideways glance he had done earlier after speaking to Benny Schmalz.

She shrugged.

'You know him?'

'I don't know anyone.'

Guy stood waiting.

'Why's he giving us the tent?' he said again.

'Because we need one. It's going to rain soon.'

He looked up at the sky and grunted in agreement.

'What have you done?'

'I haven't done anything. I never do anything. You know me,' she appealed to him.

He looked at her, wanting to be reassured, but unconvinced.

Guy knelt down so that he was on eyelevel with them.

Aida made a point of not looking at him, fingering her T-shirt instead and thinking that soon she'd be able to wash it.

He was trying to speak, but she didn't understand a word he was saying. What she did understand, however, was that his hands were shaking, and he wanted them to take the tent.

'Maybe we're just lucky,' she said to her father.

'We're never lucky.' He picked at something between his teeth. 'Soon as you think you're lucky, you stop thinking.'

She was inclined to agree with him – as they often did on most things – and didn't say anything.

Guy got slowly to his feet, looking down at the tent.

Aida stared at his boots again.

'I want the tent,' she said quietly.

Her father didn't say anything, but she knew he'd heard. He put his hands in his pockets. A pose. A stance. Then he slowly nodded.

The man hesitated.

Her father stared at him.

The man stared down at the tent as if he had expected more out of it, then walked slowly away.

'He'll be back,' her father said, as sure of himself as if he was talking about the weather.

Aida ignored him, cautiously pulling the tent towards her.

David sat out on the balcony, half-heartedly rebuking himself for not watering the dying spider plant in the corner. As the last of a day-long convoy passed – an armoured car flying a small French flag – the road audibly exhaled. He got up from the plastic chair and went back into the apartment.

Sophia's mother was still sitting in front of the TV.

On the table in the living room there was a large bouquet of flowers wrapped in cellophane with red and white hearts printed on it, and a ceramic teddy bear hanging from the bow. They had been there since he got back from the Rudinskis' residence.

'She's marvellous, isn't she?' Mrs Kačakova said.

David made out Joan Collins on the screen.

'Marvellous for her age. A wonderful woman.' She swivelled round in her chair. 'Going out?'

Before he had time to answer there was a bang from upstairs. The chandelier hanging above the table started shaking and let out a wary tinkling sound. Then there was yelling.

'Could you turn the TV up?'

He walked over and pressed the switch. Joan Collins came up close. He glanced out of the window then back at the screen.

'You want to know who those flowers are from?' Mrs Kačakova

said suddenly. She kept her eyes trained on the screen. 'We haven't got a big enough vase for them.' She started to chuckle.

David looked at the bucket the bouquet was ungraciously balanced in.

'There's a love story behind those flowers. A great love story.' She sounded very self-satisfied as she said this.

He thought she was going to say something else, but she didn't. She turned her full attention back to admiring Joan Collins.

He went into the sitting room, slamming the doors behind him so that the glass panes rattled.

When he left the apartment at 8. 00 p.m., Sophia's mother and two of her elderly neighbours were sitting on deckchairs among the cacti in the hallway, shaking their heads like a pack of retired statesmen over the NATO bomb that had hit the Chinese embassy in Belgrade.

They stopped talking when he appeared, and as he started down the stairs he heard the elderly women break into laughter. Their laughter sounding disconcertingly like the laughter of young girls.

He headed out of the block, along Ulida Odredi and on to Boulevard Partisanska, towards the city centre. When he got there, the main square was as usual resounding with the crackle of bangers, scattered across the cobblestones by groups of boys. The square itself was a minefield, and people who had unwittingly made their way into it had to find a way out and so were reduced to crossing the cobblestones bent double, trying to make out the pellets before their feet made contact with them. The scene provoked endless wonder and hysteria in the perpetrators standing beneath the trees.

He remembered the square at Christmas with its towering fir tree, the first time he came to the Republic. As the wind from the river blew the top of the tree from side to side the blue light from the revolving police siren strapped to its top went coursing unevenly round. At ground level, a tall spindly Father Christmas, in a rotting costume, accompanied by a reindeer with a rapidly declining will to survive had waited by a billboard, inviting children to have their photographs taken.

He walked slowly towards the old bank, now a club, where he was meant to be meeting Sophia, guessing he'd reached it by the high volume of bouncers at the door.

Inside, the original warren of rooms had been kept, each one decorated in a different colour with different murals painted on the walls. The themes varied but the ornate, detailed lewdness didn't.

He worked his way through a maze of corridors. The rooms he peered into were all crowded and dimly lit. There was a blue room full of badly dressed internationals; a room full of men in suits, and rooms with mostly girls in – seriously got-up girls wearing plenty of jewelled accessories for what light there was to reflect off.

There was no sign of Sophia.

He eventually found the bar in a room painted red, slightly larger than the rest, and made his way rapidly through a bloody Mary.

The club was clearly a crossroads for government dignitaries and dignitaries from the alternative state of organised crime.

He was half-way through his second bloody Mary when Sophia arrived wearing a shiny white shirt that was such a fusion of manmade fibres, he instinctively moved his cigarette away.

She sat down on the stool next to him, their knees briefly touching, and ordered herself a vodka.

After the first few sips, she examined the plum-coloured lip-stain on the side of the glass and shook her head.

'You're late,' David said.

'After all these years, I get to be late. You know that.' She opened a new pack of cigarettes and put it on the bar between them.

'How's the writing going?'

'The writing?' He hunched his shoulders and laughed. 'This afternoon I sat in the apartment with the Dictaphone whirring and a pen in my hand – thinking about my obituary. That's how it's going – not unusual at the moment.'

They ordered a bottle of wine and moved to one of the tables against the far wall where there were reproductions of the Republic's most famous icons. David had a smaller copy of the one they sat under in his London flat.

'Your last few articles have been pretty shit,' Sophia said, pouring them a glass of wine each.

David nodded in agreement.

'You come across as this tiny civilised thing trying to find its way into the middle of a war. Any war.'

He nodded again.

Neither of them said anything for a while.

'I'm glad you read them.'

She ignored this. 'I'm still trying to work out what you're doing here. Haven't you got anywhere else to go?'

He smiled. He liked her hardness. It was the most honest thing about her.

'You know I've got nowhere else to go.'

'What are you trying to do – make me feel sorry for you?'

She looked at him then looked away.

People pushing into the bar now had wet hair and clothes.

'It's raining,' David said, automatically.

Sophia watched the people trying to cram into the room. 'It's allowed to, isn't it?'

'I suppose,' he conceded, uncertain. The fact of rain unsettled him. It hadn't rained since his arrival in the Republic. 'You know what a man who doesn't make compromises is?'

'What?'

'A failure.'

'Who told you that?'

'My father.'

He watched, unsure whether she believed him or not. She often chose not to believe him.

She poured out the rest of the bottle. 'You want another one – something from Ohrid?' She called the waiter.

David watched her place her hand on the man's arm.

'The first compromise you make, you feel good, like a grown-up. By the second one you realise – very quickly – that there's not much point in growing up.'

'What did you do – kill somebody?' she asked.

'Not with my bare hands. But I know that I've been indirectly responsible for the deaths of people – many times.'

'Nobody stays clean – those who do, don't survive.'

'So you agree with my father then?'

'Look around you . . . I've taken bribes from at least half the people here. Others I've negotiated with and others I've refused. I don't have a method – I go through phases. I just want to see my country do well – get well. I hate to disappoint you, but neither of us is a bad person.'

'That's the whole difference though – you compromise with

113

motive. I compromise without.' He was about to add something else when he saw a young man making his way over to their table.

Sophia stood up. 'Tomo.'

David watched her and the young man exchange a kiss. The young man let his hand rest in the small of her back and when he bought it away the fabric of her suit jacket was creased. She was the same height as him.

'What are you doing here?'

'My parents are arguing – I couldn't stand the noise any longer.'

'Tomo lives on Floor Twelve – the floor above us.'

Tomo nodded at David. 'Is he the foreigner sleeping on your sofa?'

'The foreigner?' She looked at David, who didn't respond. He was too busy trying to work out which word offended him most: 'foreigner' or 'sofa'.

'Do you want to join us?' Sophia asked.

'No, I'm with someone.'

She pushed her head back slightly and stared with interest at the table he was pointing to.

'Which one?'

'Which one do you think?'

He watched Sophia take a good look at Violetta, in her over-sized clothes, and the American woman, Angie Fisk, from World Refugee Council.

'The one on the right. The manic depressive.'

Tomo smiled.

'Only you're not with her yet, are you?' Sophia said with an easy smile of her own. 'You're just hanging in there.'

'At least I'm not with the American.'

'You wouldn't be.'

'Why's that?'

She shrugged.

He pulled her towards him and whispered something in her ear. Then turned round and, with a small wave, headed back to his own table.

'Is that how you treat all young offenders you work with?'

'He's not a young offender – I told you. He lives in the apartment above mine. I've known him since he was this high.'

'Children grow.' David glanced over at Tomo's table and poured himself another glass of wine. 'What did he say to you?'

'He said he wouldn't be with the American because he doesn't like foreigners.'

David tried to sit back, to effect a slouch, but the bar was packed and someone had their hands on the back of his chair.

'I think he said "we" don't like foreigners,' he said, giving up trying to slouch and leaning forwards instead, aware that he wasn't holding things together in the way he wanted.

'OK, he did say "we" don't like foreigners. It's true – you know I'm racist.'

She finished her glass of wine and looked around her at the crowded bar.

'He also said it's because we prefer to make love in our own language.'

John Rudinski sat at his desk with the phone against his ear, listening to it ring; listening to it not being picked up.

If he went home now, he'd find her asleep on the sofa . . . the TV on . . . the last spilt drink staining the carpet. Or she might just have made it upstairs where, if it was beginning to get dark, she would have taken her sleeping pills. Because she didn't like the dark. And if she'd taken the sleeping pills before 8.00 p.m., she'd be up at 4.00 a.m. the next morning, unable to sleep. She'd switch all the lights in the house on, go downstairs and start making a three-course breakfast. Then he'd have to go down and eat pancakes at 4.30 a.m. and pretend it was 7.30 a.m. She'd say that the embassy car was late coming for him and he'd agree. She'd go to the front door and check to see that it hadn't pulled up on the drive.

He'd tell her not to worry, to go back to bed.

The smile would fade and she'd admit defeat. Go back upstairs, take another pill and fall back asleep until 11.00 a.m. By which time he'd be sitting back at this desk waiting for Helen, his secretary, to put through Ellen who would be hysterical because she'd woken up to find herself alone.

He pressed the recall button on his phone one last time, counted ten dial tones then put it down.

'Helen!' he called out.

He heard the squeak of her chair as she wheeled it over to the doorway.

She had her spectacles on. This always unnerved him.

'I wonder if you could help me.'

'I've got a stack of . . .'

'No,' he almost shouted. 'I want a recommendation – that's all.' He paused. 'Do you know a good place to go out?'

She took her spectacles off and stared at him.

'I mean a bar – just a bar or some place?'

'I do know of one good bar – by reputation only. I've never made it past the bouncers.'

'Oh.'

She shifted in her chair and it let out a squeak.

'Do you have an address?'

She carried on staring at him and it occurred to Rudinski that his secretary thought he might be hitting on her.

'Sure,' she said with a quick smile. 'I'll draw you a map. It's OK,' she added.

He heard her pen scratching out directions.

'Here. Don't forget to tell me what it's like,' she called out after him.

He gave his driver the name of the bar.

The driver seemed to know it, and took him there without a question.

They pulled up opposite the city's new McDonald's.

Rudinski got out the car. For once he made a clean exit without getting any of his clothing caught on anything. He stood on the kerbside for a while, feeling the roof of the car under the palm of his hand.

'You want me to wait?' the driver asked.

The air wasn't cold despite it being dark and only May. Rudinski suddenly knew what he was going to do. He took one last sniff at the night.

'No,' he said, getting back in the car. 'I want you to take me home.'

Out of her right eye, Violetta watched Angie Fisk, the overweight American, straighten her hair. Out of her left, she watched Tomo make his way back to their table. The woman he had been speaking to was also watching him.

Tomo sat down.

'Who was that?'

'A neighbour. Lives in the apartment below ours.'

Violetta knew the question she wanted to ask, and also knew she couldn't ask it.

'She once stopped me from emigrating.'

He turned back to Angie Fisk and within minutes was talking to her about American movies she hadn't seen and should have.

'There's this part in *Wag the Dog* where Dustin Hoffman – he's great at this – says, "I know what we need – we need a war." And De Niro – he's going along with this – he says, "Where're we going to get a war from? Who are we going to go to war with?" Well, this stumps Hoffman for a bit, but then he comes out with it. "I know," he says, "Albania." De Niro turns to him, confused, and says, "Albania? Where's that?" and Hoffman goes, "Precisely."'

Angie Fisk laughed. She didn't know whether she was being set up or not, but she laughed anyway. 'I'll have to see that.'

'It's a great movie,' Tomo said.

Angie Fisk turned out to be an avid collector of Bruce Lee movies – even admitted to going on line to track down rare memorabilia. Violetta listened as Angie told Tomo stuff he'd never dreamt of knowing about Bruce Lee. She didn't join in; she felt happy just to sit and listen.

Tomo was good with strangers. Good at beginnings. She wondered how he was at keeping things running . . . at finishing things. Beginnings and endings evaded her. They were symptomatic of natural, finite life and she'd spent too much time with numbers – in the universe at large – to really understand life on earth.

She had been of the opinion – from a very early age – that all finite things, including people, were essentially dishonest because they knew that at some point they had began and at some point they must end. Under such circumstances, what could people do but become dishonest? Any search for truth was nothing more than a stab at trying to claim an understanding – no matter how small – of the infinite.

Angie Fisk was laughing again.

That was another thing Tomo was good at – making people laugh. He didn't know it, but he was.

Violetta, who knew nothing about martial arts or Bruce Lee, sat patiently waiting for them to run out of things to say – or to change the subject. Which they soon did when Angie Fisk asked them if they recognised the man in the V-neck sweater three tables away – the *America Worldwide* reporter Harvey Mauser.

David and Sophia were looking at the same thing: Harvey Mauser in casual, without his mac or his microphone, sitting opposite a young Albanian girl.

'Something's eating away at him. Looks like he's got an appendicitis,' Sophia said.

David slid his arms over the table, his shirt sleeves soaking up the spilt wine. 'Or he's going to cry.'

'He's the sort of man who says exactly the wrong thing in bed at exactly the wrong moment. That's what she's thinking. No, in fact she's not even thinking it, she knows it.' Sophia paused and turned to David. 'What's he thinking?'

'He's not. He wants her. That's all.'

'Does he know he wants her?'

'Oh, he knows.'

Sophia watched the girl tuck her hair behind her ear.

David said, 'Who wouldn't?' Then he paused. 'The point is whether she wants him. He knows that's the point as well.'

'She could have him for breakfast.'

'That's something else he knows. But the overriding feeling is the wanting – he hasn't wanted anything in a very long time.'

They watched Harvey Mauser order another round, and Flora scan the bar.

'How does he do it?' David said, shaking his head. 'He's all broken up yet he's sitting there looking immaculate. He's even got a suntan for fuck's sake . . . how d'you manage to get a suntan between here and the Aleksandar Palace?'

Sophia rubbed her fingers up and down the side of the wine glass.

'He reminds me of the woman I spent this morning with,' David continued.

'Who was that?'

'The American Vice-Ambassador's wife.'

'What was she like?'

'Broken. Only she didn't hide it as well.'

'Did you think of mending her?'

'I don't know. I couldn't make my mind up.'

David thought about the back garden stretching out behind the hillside villa. About Ellen Rudinski curled up on the sun lounger, convalescing without the excuse of being an invalid. Then he thought about the woman next door standing waiting in the open doorway in her peach kimono, and how he never wanted someone else's wife in a peach kimono waiting for him in any doorway anywhere in the world.

He leant suddenly across the table again, soaking his shirt sleeves a second time.

'Who are the flowers from?' he asked.

'What flowers?' Sophia's face was open – smiling.

'There's a bouquet in your apartment. Sorry to spoil the surprise.'

'A bouquet?'

'A fucking great big one – and I know it's not from your boyfriend.'

'How do you know that?'

'Because I don't want to think you're in love with someone who sends you a bouquet wrapped in cellophane with hearts all over it and a teddy bear hanging from it.'

'I told you – I'm not in love.'

He watched her face get harder.

'What's the date today?' she asked.

'May 7th?'

'You want to know about that bouquet? The woman upstairs, she's been getting a bouquet like that for twenty years. Every May 7th for the past twenty years. Think about that.'

'The bouquet's hers?'

'The man who sent it proposed to her twenty years ago today. She turned him down, but every year she gets that bouquet, and every year it ends up in our apartment. The woman's Tomo's mother.'

David looked back over at the young man talking to the over-weight American.

'Does he know?'

Sophia shook her head.

'Who's the man?'

'The Managing Director of Republika Foods.'

She picked up the wine bottle and tried to pour herself another glass, but it was empty. So she lit a cigarette instead.

'I asked your mother about the flowers. She said that there was a love story behind them.'

'She did? Well, she was right.'

'But she didn't say that they weren't yours.'

Smiling, Sophia said, 'Maybe she likes to think somebody was sending them to me. That way she doesn't have to feel sorry for me always being on the tail end of somebody else's love story.'

'It must have rained earlier,' Violetta said, looking at the wet pavement outside the bar.

'You want to go to Flux? It's still early.'

She shook her head. 'You go.'

Tomo didn't say anything and they carried on walking together.

After a while the boulevard started to run alongside the municipal park and they turned left into the trees.

They walked in silence, every now and then one of them stepping on the night's debris of syringes that crunched underfoot. They heard the noises of animals and humans, making the most of the ten hours of darkness, but didn't see anything.

Without flower-beds or any other signs of cultivation, the park had always felt more like a clearing in a forest. The only things to break up the wilderness were the hard-nosed statues of heroes from Tito's Yugoslavia, which had been repeatedly vandalised and repaired, and were now too overgrown for even the vandals to find.

The Republic's new football stadium marked the park's western boundary and they soon reached the arc of light stretching into the trees from the stadium's floodlights.

'That's better,' Tomo said.

'Were you afraid?'

'No – I just don't like walking in parks at night – it's not safe.'

'No, it's not safe,' she agreed.

'So what do you want to do?'

'This – just this. Walking with you.'

'There are other places we could walk.'

She was a few paces ahead of him, the light from the stadium streaking across her back, when something came out of the trees, flying low at them.

The air was suddenly full of heavy squawking.

'What's that?'

'Parakeets,' Violetta said.

Tomo laughed.

'You don't believe me? People have them as pets – get bored of them, or they escape. They've been breeding in the park for over a decade, slowly adapting to our climate and eating the smaller birds whose natural habitat this is.'

The squawking started again and this time Tomo saw bright green among the trees.

They stopped to look.

'It doesn't sound natural.'

'There's no reason why a piece of Brazilian rainforest should. Here.'

She started to move away from the tree with the parakeets in.

'They look even stranger in winter. In the snow.'

'You come here in the winter?'

'A lot.'

'So walking in parks in the dark is another thing you're not afraid of?'

'What d'you mean by that?'

She stopped, waiting for him to catch up with her.

'I mean that I've got a list as long as my arm of things that don't frighten you, but I still don't know of a single thing that does.'

Violetta didn't say anything, staring through the broken wire fence they'd come to at the old fairground among the trees.

'I used to come here.'

The only thing still standing was the carousel, whose carriages – although piebald with rust – were otherwise intact.

'The woman who operated it had no teeth.'

Tomo looked over at the blue plastic kiosk next to the carousel and thought he remembered the door opening and a woman with a toothless grin emerging. But this might have been Violetta's memory, not his.

'Sometimes I'm afraid,' Violetta said, not looking at him, her fingers threaded through the wire mesh fence. 'I'm afraid now.'

He watched her unthread her fingers and study the flakes of rust on them.

'I thought the park at night was something you're not afraid of?'

'Right now I'm afraid of not being in the park. I'm afraid of going back to my apartment.'

He turned towards her.

'What are we doing here?'

'We're standing looking at a carousel in a disused fairground because I'm afraid of going back to my apartment with you where we'll end up fucking.'

'I never did like the carousel.'

'I knew I couldn't trust you.'

Tomo's mother sat out on the balcony listening to her husband's grunting laughter through the open door. She'd left him slumped on the sofa watching TV, his gut shaking as he laughed the only laughter in his repertoire: the sort that celebrated the misfortune of others. Probably provoked by the sight on screen of the Chinese embassy in Belgrade going up in smoke.

They'd argued earlier. He said that all her questions sounded like accusations and she said that he had no ideals.

She wrapped her cardigan around her and, balancing her feet in their slippers on the bottom of the railing, leant forward and watched Sophia and her foreigner make their way up the street.

A few minutes later she heard the door to their building banging shut.

She went back into the lounge. Her husband was asleep, his head lolling rhythmically to one side. Her embroidery had fallen to the floor. Picking it up, she switched off the TV and went back outside on to the balcony.

She could hear the TV now from Sophia's apartment, and smelt smoke curling up from the downstairs balcony. The foreigner did the same thing every night.

The smell of smoke disappeared. There was a faint sigh, followed by the scraping of the plastic chair as he got up. The balcony door was shut and the wooden shutters clattered down.

She went and stood against the railings, watching the empty street below. The streetlights reflecting in the puddles.

After about ten minutes, a figure appeared walking up the middle of the road, head down, hands in pockets.

Something stopped her calling out to Tomo. She just stayed pressed against the railings, watching him. Boris had told her about Violetta Nebkov. Told her what he thought about Tomo and Violetta Nebkov.

Tomo hadn't said anything to her about the girl, but she'd seen how it was with him.

That's why tonight she hadn't expected him to come back

home. Hadn't expected to see him walking up the middle of the road, head down.

She listened to her husband's snoring, which had replaced the grunting laughter, and thought she was going to start screaming at the top of her voice. She closed her eyes.

You're telling yourself that you're only twenty-six . . . you think there'll be other nights like this. She opened her eyes and stared down at her slippers, which were fraying at the toes. But there won't. There'll never be another night like this ever again and you know it.

In the street below, Tomo stopped in his tracks. He took his hands out of his pockets, letting them hang loosely down by his sides.

He turned around, caught for a second in the headlights of a purple Yugo trying to park.

The headlights went dim and he started walking rapidly away from the block, back in the direction he had just come from, until he turned on to the main boulevard and out of sight.

He was gone. It was starting to rain again and the road was empty. This fact suddenly struck her as unbearable.

24 °c

14 May 1999 / First ICRC explorative mission to Kosovo since its withdrawal on 29 March

Donatella stood in the centre of the room watching Fatos as he attempted to install the rows of new computers, and Valbona as she methodically loaded the software. She watched them both in a detached way. They were only three weeks behind schedule and the rest of the money for completion of the community centre was now in place. The computers, tables and chairs had – miraculously – arrived to order, yet she stood watching the young actor, Fatos, and Valbona, feeling nothing but the creeping onset of apathy.

She recognised the apathy as a symptom of exhaustion, and gave into it, only just managing to rouse herself when Guy Spiers walked into the room.

'What's with the queue outside?' he asked.

'The promise of internet access – how long is it?'

'Way down past the mosque. Almost at Petri's.'

She made a mental note to get a picture of the queue for her report – *refugees queue for internet access at new community centre.*

'The lorry arrived yesterday and we're already one terminal short – stolen before they'd even started unloading. We found the driver lying in the back with one glove on and a wound to the head – he'd been concussed with a plank of wood.'

'Refugees or people from the village?'

'No idea.' She let herself sink back under the weight of exhaustion. 'There's a locksmith coming this afternoon to fit locks

124

into doors that – this morning – the carpenter informed me won't be ready for another week. So now I'm stuck trying to arrange twenty-four-hour security for the computers that haven't been stolen. Yet.'

'It's looking good in here,' he said.

'Yeah, it's looking good,' Donatella conceded, aware that he was trying to soothe. 'But we still don't have a roof.'

They watched Fatos and Valbona working, in syncopation, on separate things.

'Did you ever find out where the circus tent came from?' she said after a while.

'Romania. That poor guy was speaking Romanian. Not even Howard picked up on it.'

Donatella didn't say anything – she wasn't interested in Romania.

'I wanted to talk to Peter about the tent. The community centre's grand opening is planned for the beginning of June some time and I was wondering if Peter would organise getting the tent erected to coincide with this – maybe have a party?' She paused, turning to Fatos. 'It would be a great place to have a party, wouldn't it?'

Fatos smiled, but was too shy to speak. He turned intently back to the length of cable he was holding.

'It would make a great theatre as well – the circus tent. What was the play the professor wanted to do?'

'*Julius Caesar*,' Fatos mumbled. Then, looking up, 'We can make village theatre?'

'I'll speak to the professor.'

Fatos nodded, and took hold of the cable once more.

Donatella asked Guy for a pen and scribbled *Julius Caesar* across her hand.

Guy watched the biro maul her skin, preoccupied.

'I wanted to ask you about English lessons.'

'Here at the centre?'

He nodded.

'They're pretty much full up. Whoever it is better put their name down. You should speak to Valbona – she takes the lessons. Wait,' she said as Guy made his way towards Valbona, hunched over a computer screen with her back to them. 'Is your friend David still in the country?'

'David? I think so.'

'I thought he might want to come to the Mayor's meal tonight – I'm sure the presence of a journalist would flatter Mr Berisha's ego.'

The air in the old cinema was full of sawdust and asbestos and the sunlight that made its way into the building was filthy. At the back, near the door, there was a stove surrounded by charred logs, left over from whatever activities it had been lit to warm in the winter months. Protruding at regular intervals along the walls on either side of the room were bunches of wires – relics from the cinema's brief career as a shoe factory. At the far end there was an imposing proscenium arch stage.

As Spatim walked across the floor the old blanket nailed to the wall on his right moved to one side and Balon and Lirije, the Mayor's daughter, appeared in the doorway the blanket had concealed.

Spatim watched Lirije accept the two cans of potted meat Balon took out of his pocket – an idiot's gift. She accepted them graciously then made her way over to him.

Balon's face broke into a grin, then, after staring morosely at his feet for a while, he disappeared back behind the old blanket. He'd only gone as far as the other room where the shoes and potted meat were kept, but that didn't matter.

Spatim climbed awkwardly on to the stage, pulling Lirije up after him. They went into the wings where there was an enormous projector, still intact, and where they couldn't be seen from the auditorium if anyone came in. He unfolded the rug they kept there and sat down.

They risked a cigarette between them because there was so much dust anyway that anyone coming in wouldn't detect the smoke. He sat with his knees up and his arms balanced on them because he was wearing a sleeveless T-shirt and his arms looked best like this. When he looked at her she looked straight back.

He glanced at the two tins of potted meat then leant forward and stroked the side of her neck. Sometimes she brushed his hand with her ear, but she didn't today. She just smiled at him and kept her distance.

She never bored him with the details of any personal torment she might suffer as a result of their secret meetings. He didn't know if she ever felt guilty – he guessed not.

What he did know was that, for the first time in his life, he'd made the mistake of telling a girl that he loved her — and meant it. He'd poured himself at her feet, felt more light-headed than he'd ever done during Ramadan, and had got nothing in return. She had just stared down at him in silence, and it was almost as if she knew that the effect of her silence made him believe the words he had spoken. If she'd spoken herself at that moment, he might not have, but now he was stuck with this immense belief ... this immense sense of faith he had never experienced before — not even sure it was rightfully his.

'I haven't got long,' she said, reminding him. 'The meal at the house tonight.' Then, after a while, 'Make me laugh.'

He stared down at his boots, wiping the dust off the leather.

'We're sitting above enough ammunition to start our own war.'

'I'm not laughing.'

He looked up at her then looked back down at his boots, unsure of himself today.

'I don't know — you might not find it funny.' He hesitated. 'I could tell you something about a friend of mine in London.'

'London?' she said, as if she had no intention of finding it funny.

'I think it was London,' he said. It was always like this when she asked him a question; he immediately started to doubt himself.

'My friend, he worked for this woman, cleaning.'

Lirije nodded, waiting.

'She was a rich woman.'

He watched her take this in.

'You know what she had him do? She had him do all the ironing — naked.'

She didn't laugh; it was Spatim who was laughing. What he said made her thoughtful. 'Did he make much money?'

'Lots of money.'

She started picking at a loose button on her jacket.

'If we were in London would you do that? The ironing job?'

'Of course — some rich woman's stupid enough and lonely enough to pay me to take my clothes off and do her ironing — course.'

She nodded to herself. 'Good.'

He sat there thinking that he never knew what she was going to say next.

She got to her feet brushing herself down.

'Got to get back before I'm missed. Balon!' she called out.

'I had to see you today,' he said suddenly, urgently, trying to catch hold of her hand.

'Balon,' she called out again. Then, turning back to Spatim, 'It's not fair,' she said, kicking his boot. 'You were supposed to make me laugh and instead I end up making you laugh.' She paused. 'You owe me.'

He stayed up on the stage as she jumped down. Wondering why fate decreed that the easiest thing in the world was asking a girl you didn't love to spend time with you in a motel room, and the hardest thing in the world to ask one you did.

The sun had moved round so that it was directly above Aida where she was sitting staring at the threadbare grass and the way the tent pegs had bent in the hard ground. Her T-shirt was now clean, but had shrunk a size when she washed it, which had made her cry.

She got up and went inside the tent, out of the sun.

Her father had just finished his ready meal. The yellow carton lay empty and discarded underneath the camp bed, like something he felt guilty for having partaken of. His jaw hung slack and he was running his tongue over his teeth to get rid of the taste.

He eyed her briefly then went back to staring at the tent floor, shifting his feet more widely apart to let a belch rise and grimacing as the taste of the meal repeated on him. He nodded at her bed where he knew she kept a packet of cigarettes, and watched as she took the packet out from under the pillow then put it back.

As he started to smoke, his face relaxed.

They both had too many secrets to talk any more, so it surprised her when he said, 'We're going to America.'

He said it without looking up, and after saying it started slowly nodding to himself.

She sat down on the camp bed opposite him, thinking.

When he did at last look up, he gave her one of those puzzled stares. As if she was the one who had just spoken and not him. He'd been looking at her like this ever since she could remember – trying to work out whether he hated her or not.

She'd tried to make it easier for him by hating him back, and had only ever once thought of loving him. He had been crossing the courtyard at home holding a cheese in his hand and trying not

128

to trip up in the mud – which was difficult, not only because he was slightly bow-legged, but because at that time of year the mud stuck like glue – and he had looked up, seen her face through the kitchen window, and smiled.

Her father with the cheese and the smile was like the moment with her mother and the tomatoes. Moments which, in themselves, felt whole.

She stared at him now, not knowing what to feel. 'How?'

He didn't respond.

'You need visas for America.'

Nodding, he said, 'We'll buy visas.'

'How?' she said again.

'With money.'

This was the sticking point. They didn't have any money. But she could tell from his face that this wasn't gong to be an obstacle; that he had a plan and this plan was his secret.

'I've never seen the sea before,' he said, stubbing his cigarette out carefully and putting the stub in his pocket.

She didn't know he'd ever given the sea any thought. 'Are we going by boat?'

'No – aeroplane. We'll see the sea from the aeroplane.'

She paused. 'I don't want to go to America – I've got other plans.'

He looked up sharply. 'We're going to America,' he repeated firmly, getting to his feet with a grunt, his head at an angle because the tent wasn't tall enough for him to stand up straight in.

She thought he was going to get angry, like he used to with her mother when he would end up shouting at her that he deserved to be feared, that, after everything, this was his due – the least he deserved.

Aida watched now as his neck took the strain, and heavy breathing flecked his chin with spittle.

Then, just at the moment when she thought he was going to strike, he changed tack and let go of it all. The tautness went. He sagged and no longer had to bow his head to fit in the tent.

'Has it ever occurred to you that I'm an old man?'

This was a new approach. Why didn't he hit her? It had cost him a lot not to, and she had the feeling that he hadn't because it would ruin his plan in some way.

'I don't want to die in this place.'

129

She didn't quibble over whether he was telling the truth or not – this was for him to know. What interested her was the fact that he was appealing to a sense of compassion he wasn't even sure she had.

Pushing him, she said, 'But you don't mind dying in America?'

The tent was just about big enough at night, when they were both – for some of the time anyway – unconscious. But after an exchange like this it was definitely too small. One of them would have to go and her father – already on his feet – pulled the flap back and stepped outside.

David wished the phone wasn't in the hallway. He liked to have a view while speaking on the phone, but the only thing he could see from Sophia's hallway was a toilet with a yellow pipe stuck down it – now used as an outlet for the water from the washing machine.

He stood listening to the dial tones with his right ear and the pigeons scratching on the outside of the toilet window ledge with his left.

'Sally – it's David.'

'David? Where in the world are you?'

He knew – as soon as she said this – that she was going to put whatever she was doing in her office at *Geographica* to one side and give him some time.

'Here. Still here. How's life in Washington?'

'Life in Washington's life in Washington.'

At fifty-seven, Sally knew what she was talking about. She was a first-generation female white-collar worker, and had been one of a kind when she started to travel on commuter trains in the days when – as she put it – gentlemen used to give up their seats. This was the great dividing line for her between the world then and the world now, and marked a genuine decline in civilisation. The latterday female executives and those who had risen far above the ranks thought nothing of her, but she knew she was one of the pioneers who had built their world. Sally had been there at the beginning – a precursor of the world as they knew it.

'Is Robert around?'

'Since when have you wanted to speak to Robert?'

She had known as soon as she picked up the phone why he was calling. But she wasn't going to let him say that he was no longer writing . . . that he couldn't write. She didn't want him to hear himself say it.

'I don't know what I'm doing here.'

'Then write that up . . . that you don't know what the hell you're doing there.'

Thousands of miles away, he heard someone enter Sally's office; heard her rattling around in her pencil tub and her lucky-charm bracelet scraping against the keyboard.

Suddenly afraid, he said, 'I'll let you go.'

'David – wait. You've got to start making promises to yourself and you've got to start keeping them. You need your words – I need your words.'

'Sally,' he reprimanded her.

Later on he left the apartment, skidding in pools of water from where Sophia's mother had watered the cactii earlier.

Outside the breeze had dropped.

Summer was beginning and the city knew it.

Driving out towards Stengova, he passed a K-For convoy and a lorry with a prefabricated village on its back. At the toll, just before the turn-off, he hit another traffic jam caused by a Yugo this time.

He got out of his car and walked up to the Yugo at the head of the queue, which had four redneck Texans in it.

'Something happening?' he asked, eyeing the coffin strapped to the roof of the car and the nearby group of police.

'Already happened – Jerry died.'

One of the backseat Texans added, with a strong sense of injustice, 'Signed on to help re-build roads into Kosovo. Jerry died on the job – heart attack.'

A policeman turned to watch David talking to the Texans.

'We made a coffin, nailed Jerry up in it, then put him on the roof of the car. Now we're waiting for somebody from the embassy to arrive. It's illegal to take a body out of the country it's died in – never knew that,' the Yugo's driver said in a slow drawl.

'We were en route for the airport,' someone from the back seat put in. 'Jerry's still got the other half of a return ticket – we were kind of hoping to get him on a plane tonight.'

The driver, nodding his head, added, 'He's got family back home, waiting to bury him.'

David, thinking this made sense, said, 'Well, I hope Jerry makes his flight.'

Eventually the queue of traffic managed to get past the jam caused by the four living and one dead Texan.

David's car passed through the tolls then turned off the main road. The Fiat was soon covered in dust.

Half an hour later, he parked the car at the Women Against War HQ, and headed for the camp in search of Donatella.

The first person he saw was Howard, pushing his hands through his hair and shouting loudly at a group of local men.

A trio of well-dressed men and women made their way over to a group of reluctant children Nadia and Giulietta were attempting to coax into a line.

A man standing nearby turned and slapped David's hand. 'Lay me five,' he said with a grin.

'I'm impressed,' David smiled back.

'Lay me five,' the man said again, with the same grin.

'What's your name?'

'Lay me five.'

Realising that this was the only reply to any direct questions he was going to get, David watched with relief as Howard made his way over.

'You here for the Mayor's dinner?' he asked.

David nodded, unsure whether this pleased Howard or not.

The man started talking rapidly in Albanian.

'They want his children,' Howard announced after several minutes.

'Lay me five,' the man piped up.

'Who wants them?'

'They do.'

Howard turned and pointed to the trio now milling around the children.

'For a photo shoot. I think Hillary Clinton's coming, and they want children she can have her photograph taken with. Beautiful children.'

The man went off to find his children with a last, 'Lay me five'.

They found Donatella at the Italian stew kitchen.

'You came,' she said, looking up at David.

He liked her for making it sound like he had a choice; that he might have something else to do.

'So, the Clintons are coming?' he said, sitting down opposite her.

'Apparently. One of them, anyway.' She stood up. 'I'd better go and get the kids ready for the next beauty parade. There's a whole load of them hiding from Nadia and Giulietta. We've got about forty-five minutes,' she said with a quick determined glance at her watch.

'Is Guy around?'

'Somewhere – he's difficult to find these days.'

'He's found himself a girl?' David guessed.

'He's found himself a refugee.'

'You're afraid for her?'

'No, I'm afraid for him.' She walked off with a stoop.

Harvey pushed his way round the crowded room where everybody was talking and nobody was listening, giving a mouth-stretching smile whenever he was recognised. He managed not to speak. His head was full of smoke and raki.

The room smelt of sweat, aftershave, perfume and all the other things rooms smelt of when the people in them didn't have the courage to say what they were thinking.

This wasn't the thing he hated most though. The thing he hated most was the fact that the windows had no curtains so the only thing you could see through them – now it was getting dark – was this goddam room he was standing in all over again.

The ICRC was inside Kosovo, slowly prising her open, and although everyone was happy right now to stand around on stained carpet, surrounded by bad furniture, drinking cocktails, they were already imagining themselves several miles north of here where there was no electricity, and mass graves waiting to be discovered. Somewhere where the work of the enemy could at least be seen; where the enemy itself could at least be identified . . . where they could put their capacity for heroism to the test.

Harvey had had time, in the last few weeks, to think. Something that hadn't happened – with any severity – since he was about eighteen.

He'd worked out, for instance, that in a village where the men have been massacred, the women have run into the forest and the houses have been burnt to the ground, it is better to convey the truth rather than try to tell it. Because – unless you were there –

you can't. It's better to talk about a small girl sitting cross-legged on a piece of carpet she's rescued from her smoking home, holding her brother's shoe, than count the bodies of the dead so that this figure can be punched into your laptop along with a whole set of other ones until the truth is, as a whole, electronically digestible. It might be better to take the trouble to find out the small girl's name − her full name − and whether the shoe she's holding, the one that got stuck on a corner of carpet before her brother was dragged away, is his left shoe or his right shoe.

He reached the bar and ordered himself another glass of the hard liquor, unable to drink the champagne being carried around on trays to celebrate the verification of ethnic cleansing.

People were laughing, having a good time. He allowed himself to call it a party. Even Flora − who sat in her apartment most nights watching *Sunset Boulevard* while waiting for the phone to ring and for it to be her parents in Priština phoning to let her know they were still alive − even she was smiling. Part of the party.

He watched her understanding about 50 per cent of what the Northern Irish journalist was saying to her, smiling anyway and letting him lay his hand on her arm.

'What are you drinking?'

He turned, confused, to the short woman standing next to him in a lemon suit with food stains down the left-hand lapel.

'What are you drinking?' Ellen Rudinski said again.

'Raki,' the bartender cut in, moving his whole face upward into the air as he said it and somehow managing to maintain his dignity despite the purple waistcoat and dickey bow.

'You can do me one of those,' she said, tapping a forefinger on the bar. 'I never did like champagne − gives me headaches. Terrible headaches.' She turned to Harvey then looked back out across the room. The fact that they were both drinking the same thing made them complicit and they didn't have to start talking right away.

He took in the lemon suit again.

'Lemon sherbet,' Ellen said, turning suddenly to him. 'The shade's lemon sherbet.' She took her first sip. 'They told me I looked good in it.'

'How many of them?'

'Three? Four?'

'I can imagine you buying it.'

'I bought it because I never thought I'd wear it, and because . . .'

She took another sip. 'My husband likes me to shop – he thinks it's a sign of mental stability.'

'Is he here tonight?'

Ellen nodded and half-thought of making Harvey guess which one was John Rudinski. 'That one over there.' She pointed him out, flanking the American Ambassador who was standing talking – without a glass of champagne and without his tie – to Irina Yupovič.

Harvey nodded, taking things in.

'He's severely contemplating falling in love with a stranger – I don't think he's ever done that before.'

Harvey said, 'Irina Yupović. The stranger's Irina Yupović – the President's wife.'

Ellen didn't make anything of this. 'He's not even thinking about the probability of whether she'd ever love him back. Right now he's just amazed with himself.'

They were both settled comfortably at the bar, oblivious to the crowd pressing around them. The champagne had run dry and people were beginning to make their way over to the bar, totting up in their heads remaining expenses, and digging in their pockets.

'I think this might make me drunk,' Ellen Rudinski said hopefully, holding her second glass of raki up to the light.

Harvey shook his head. 'I don't know – I've been drinking it solidly for the past two weeks and . . . nothing. I mean, if anything, it brings on a sort of clarity. They say that a glass a day helps to prolong your life.'

'Prolong it? Oh, God.'

They fell silent again.

Harvey carried on watching Flora, still talking to the Irishman who was probably giving her some spiel about their countries being the same size and that he knew as many terrorists as she did.

'Haven't seen you on TV the last couple of nights.'

'No – it's finished.'

'I didn't think they ran the news in series.'

He swung his head to look at her. 'I missed the storming of the embassy. You remember that – back in March?'

'I remember watching it on TV.'

'Yeah? Well, I missed it. I was covering the opening of the new McDonald's that night – giving the intro for our cameras to home in on the President taking his first bite of a McWhopper with all the shit they put inside it and that was that. One miss then you walk.'

'So you made the big Mcfuckup.' She paused. 'You told anybody yet?'

He shook his head.

'You told your wife?'

He shook his head again.

'Isn't she going to realise when she switches on and you're not there?'

'She hasn't called – she doesn't watch.'

Ellen started to laugh; a croaking laugh full of raki. 'She watches.'

'She says she doesn't.'

'That means she watches.'

'Then why hasn't she called?'

'How the hell should I know?'

They took in the room again. Harvey even took in the reflection of the room, but nothing had changed.

'Look at them all, champing at the bit. You know why that is? It's because deep down they know that history has – at this inexplicably late stage in the day – forsaken them.'

Ellen put her hand on her heart in mock relief. 'So that's what we're all doing here – looking for a piece of history in the making?'

Harvey nodded. 'Still blindly searching for it.'

Then she said, shaking her head – a genuine headshake – 'But my folks' folks were frontiers people.'

He took in the lemon sherbet suit again, for a third time – he hadn't expected this.

She'd got a hold of herself now. 'I don't need to come digging around for history in some ex-Commie shithole.'

He heard her teeth clanking on the glass and watched her drift away. They drifted out of conversation as quickly as they'd drifted in. As he slipped off the stool, he wondered briefly what she was thinking, but would never have got close to the picture Ellen Rudinski had in her head right then; one that had been haunting her ever since she'd laid eyes on it – and that was of Anne Hargreaves standing in her peach kimono in broad daylight.

He couldn't get close – although he might have done – because his field of vision was full of Flora, still talking to the midget Irishman. When he left the bar he didn't even push close past them, he headed straight for the lift and, half-drunk, found himself fumbling with the key to his room before he knew it.

He opened the door, only pausing a second before switching on the light.

There he was – reflected in the window along with everything else in Room 304. He must have been standing there for about five minutes when he saw the door behind him opening and Flora stepping hesitantly into his room.

Flora didn't know what she was doing. She'd become scared talking to the Irishman on her own. She didn't mind when she knew Harvey was watching, but she did when he left. Harvey – unlike the Irishman – didn't make her afraid.

The room smelt heavily of aftershave, soap and shampoo. It smelt cleaner than Harvey looked.

She'd been up to his room once before – when he'd printed something off his laptop that he wanted her to translate. She remembered the screensaver that came up – a photograph of his wife and daughter huddled in their anoraks at the top of a mountain in driving rain – and that she found it reassuring.

The other thing she remembered about the time they went up to his room was that she'd noticed the hem at the back of his mac had fallen down, and that the hem falling down and him not noticing it felt wrong.

She felt better already – less afraid – and allowed her jaw to work steadily again on the gum in her mouth.

At last Harvey turned round and said, 'You enjoy the party?'

'Is that what it was?' Then, giving a quick smile, she said, 'I was wondering.'

Harvey smiled back – briefly – but never lost that earnest look. Whatever the backdrop, Harvey's face somehow always managed to look earnest.

They listened to her chewing the gum.

Then she let out a sigh.

'So . . .' Harvey said.

'You left the party.'

'You were busy talking.'

'To a man from Ireland.'

'To a man from Ireland,' he agreed.

'I wanted to make sure you were still here.'

He held up his arms then let them drop back to his sides. 'I'm here – got nowhere else to go.'

She nodded slowly, still chewing.

Every now and then he saw a patch of bright pink between her teeth as she pushed the gum right to the front of her mouth.

'You're going to Kosovo?'

Now it was his turn to sigh. 'I don't know, Flora.'

She stared at him. It was the first time he'd said her name. 'Everyone else is going.'

'I know.' Now he was looking at her even more earnestly than before. 'I'm sorry,' he said, suddenly. 'What they're finding, it's . . . I mean, for you it's . . .'

She stared as blankly back at him as he was staring earnestly at her, finally locking on to each other from their opposite poles.

She was the first to break away, sitting down suddenly on the end of the bed with her back curved in the position that used to give her stomach ache when she was a child. She could almost hear her mother's voice now – here – in Room 304 at the Aleksandar Palace Hotel, scolding her about her posture. So that when the phone started suddenly ringing, for a moment she really was ready to believe that it *was* her mother, phoning from Priština to say that if she didn't sit up straight she'd get a stomach ache.

She waited for Harvey to pick up the phone and carried on staring straight ahead of her through the open bathroom door where there were puddles of water still on the floor and some toothpaste packaging that looked like it had been recently discarded. She couldn't imagine Harvey going out to buy himself things like toothpaste.

'OK, yeah, OK,' she heard him say.

Harvey stood staring at the back of Flora's head. From this angle, with her thick black hair and tiny shoulders, she looked like a young boy. The hotel room could almost have been a cabin on a ship and Flora a stowaway he had just found. He waited, without anticipation, to hear his wife's voice.

'Val? What time's it over there?'

'Around noon.'

He tried to calculate in his head, but instinctively this didn't sound right. 'Noon?'

'I'm phoning from the west coast, Harvey. We're in Seattle.' Her voice went distant as she turned her head away from the phone. 'It's raining.'

He started to panic without knowing why. 'What're you doing in Seattle?'

'Lou wanted to see her Aunt Caroline. She loves it here. Even the rain.'

She had something to tell him, he could feel it.

Flora stood up.

He moved forward and tried to grab hold of her, but the wire wasn't long enough and left his arm, full of intent, flailing around in the air just behind her.

'You really screwed up this time, Harvey. Harvey?'

'What did I do?'

Flora turned round and mouthed something at him, but he was listening to his wife, whom he couldn't see, and watching Flora, whom he couldn't hear, and each one was rendering the other useless.

'You missed Lou's birthday.'

Val was speaking low and slow. It wasn't just that he'd missed Lou's birthday, it was that he'd missed the point of missing Lou's birthday. 'Your daughter's eighteenth birthday.'

Harvey looked round the room – he was sure he'd bought her something at the bazaar. Sure. He'd forgotten to send it, that was all.

'Flora, wait,' he called out as she opened the door.

He heard Val break, starting to yell. 'Harvey? Who the fuck are you talking to, Harvey?'

Flora made her arm and hand small and gave him a minuscule wave then disappeared into the corridor, shutting the door behind her.

'Harvey, you're fucked, you know that? Completely fucked, you're . . .'

He heard his wife's voice, the fury and outrage in it, and behind her the rain in Seattle.

He turned his back on the door, facing the window instead and the reflection of the room with him standing in it, wondering why he didn't feel fucked.

As they stood waiting for Balon to open the gates to the Mayor's house, David saw that Donatella was wearing make-up and an outfit – he guessed – she kept for occasions such as these. The lapels of her jacket bore stained traces of other such functions, and her face looked like a child's. As though it had been good-naturedly smothered in the contents of her mother's make-up bag.

'Did you find Guy?'

David shook his head.

'Shame. Maybe you could have given him some advice.'

'On what?' he said. 'Happiness?'

The gates finally opened and Balon's overlarge head appeared with its lopsided features. He scraped a thick clump of black hair from his forehead to reveal wide startled eyes. Behind him stood the half-finished mayoral residence.

Balon stared for a minute at the small group of internationals standing in the road then hauled the gates back against the walls, losing his legs in a cloud of dust that reached his waist.

Despite the fact that it hadn't rained for weeks, his clothes were covered in mud.

He took them to the door of the house, but didn't go in.

They took off their shoes, putting them next to the countless other pairs on the rack then went inside. Peter Miller, Dan Hale and Spatim were already there. Spatim had to wipe his fingers, white with icing sugar from Turkish Delight, on the back of his trousers before shaking hands.

'You're the writer,' he said to David, after introducing himself. 'Maybe you write about us?'

David nodded, feeling like a huckster.

After the introductions they moved into the main room where there was about a mile of sofa covered in sheepskin rugs. The Albanian men sat down at the end near the window, and the women near the door where they talked quietly among themselves, only breaking off to stare at their guests seated in the middle.

The women were all about the same age, and looked like sisters or cousins. None of them were wearing headscarves, and David guessed that they'd been told to hang them up for the evening because of Donatella. Enver was aware that headscarves were an issue with a lot of the female humanitarians in the camp, and Donatella might have been one of them for all Enver knew. He wasn't taking any risks, and was willing to bury a lot under the carpet for the space of three hours in order to do business. They sat without speaking, the sound of children playing in an upper storey just audible above the rapid Spanish of the South American soap *Sunset Boulevard*, playing at top volume on the widescreen TV in the cabinet opposite. Every now and then the women would touch their hair.

'Where's Chris Woods?' Donatella asked Howard, who had sat down next to her.

'Didn't think the evening was high-profile enough to require his personal attendance,' Howard whispered back.

'I've been following this, it's great,' Spatim said with an appreciative nod at the TV before flicking his gaze to a girl in a Puma tracksuit who came into the room carrying a tray of Coca-Cola then disappeared again. Soon after the arrival of the Coca-Cola, all the women disappeared, one by one.

'They certainly keep the best of the crop under lock and key,' Dan Hale said benevolently, his eyes on the retreating back of the girl in the tracksuit.

'How's Guy?' David said, turning to Peter Miller, who, preoccupied, was watching Spatim watch Dan Hale.

'He's great,' he said, finally turning to David. 'Really great.'

David felt a brief blush of pride without knowing why.

'They're talking of offering me and Donatella a mission in Chechnya after all this blows over here – if Chechnya opens up that is. We were thinking of asking Guy if he wanted to come and help us run it.'

'That's fantastic. And what about Howard?'

Peter leant round David to look at Donatella and Howard further down the sofa, talking to each other. 'Howard'll go wherever Donatella goes,' he said warmly.

David found himself smiling back. Peter was one of those rare people, he realised, who reminded you of what you had, not what you didn't have, or – worse still – might never have.

'You think so?' he asked.

Peter nodded.

'I met your sister,' David said, suddenly remembering.

This surprised Peter. 'Ellen?'

David nodded. 'We met over a dead dog.' He felt that Peter deserved to know this.

'A dead dog?' Peter laughed, but didn't sound comfortable. He gave David a quick look, but didn't ask for any details. 'I'm glad,' he rounded off, not sounding any more comfortable.

Enver looked around the room at his guests. Sensing that the entertainment wasn't up to scratch, he leant forward awkwardly over his paunch and jabbed viciously at the TV controls.

'Albanian channel,' he said, as two semi-naked men standing in an apple orchard finished covering their bodies in washing-up liquid and started to wrestle.

They watched the men slide all over each other in the shade of the orchard until the door of the room opened and a woman poked her head round to say that dinner was ready. They filed into a small kitchen off the hallway, which was whitewashed and had an open staircase leading from it.

There were lots of plants and children on the stairs, who burst out laughing at the sight of them trooping into the kitchen, then disappeared back into the upper storeys.

The women didn't sit down with them. In between serving courses, they remained standing against the walls, smiling at their guests as they ate. A vast quantity of food started to emerge, miraculously, from a tiny oven: minestrone soup was followed by a bowl of stew, then a large plate of chicken, chips and rice. Seconds were offered, and couldn't be refused. Food was eaten rapidly and there was barely any conversation although the Mayor spoke occasionally to Spatim. Spatim didn't translate and seemed either not to know or to have forgotten that Howard spoke Albanian.

Eventually they staggered back into the other room. The orchard on TV, much to Peter Miller's disappointment, had vanished and the wrestlers with it. Instead, a company called Smirna Tours kept showing pictures of a Smirna Tour bus making its way along one of the Republic's motorways in the driving rain, interspersed with aerial shots of Mecca. Then a list of cut-price offers in Deutschmarks for trips to Mecca was flashed across the screen.

The women didn't reappear immediately, and when they did it was with trays of cheese, fruit, nuts, Turkish Delight and coffee.

The Mayor, anxious, switched back to *Sunset Boulevard* then leant forward to make an announcement, gesturing at Spatim to translate.

'The Mayor, he says he's very happy to have you as his guests. Great honour for him.'

'Tell him it's an honour for us also,' Donatella said, relieved to get to the point of the evening at last.

Howard nodded. Dan Hale didn't respond, his attention absorbed by *Sunset Boulevard*.

'We will never forget the work you have done here with the deportees,' Spatim continued.

'There's still much work to do,' Donatella said, quietly.

Enver's speech showed not only a flair for business acquired during Black Market days, but an unbridled appetite for civic ceremony that was the bequest of a socialist past. Despite the aura of naïvety this combination gave rise to, it had at its roots a violent lawlessness barely perceptible to the average western civilian.

David looked more closely at Enver as he said something to Spatim, gave him a brief nod to translate then got up.

'The Mayor, he apologises for state of roads. It has taken long time to raise money for tarmac. There is still a lot of mud,' Spatim said, as Enver drew a bottle of Johnnie Walker from the cabinet.

This dark corner of the cabinet concealed a great many bottles of Johnnie Walker – the result of a recent business transaction.

One of the older women brought in a tray of clean glasses and Enver poured whisky for himself, Spatim and the internationals.

'Cheers,' he said.

'The roads are our roads, not government's,' Spatim continued. 'Is same with electricity. Five years ago there was no electricity, now we have light.' He gestured towards the ceiling. 'Maybe these are things we can co-operate on.'

Howard was about to speak when Enver's father – wearing a blue cloth cap and suit jacket – walked into the room carrying a brown paper bag. He rubbed his hat backwards and forwards over his head when he laid eyes on the bareheaded women and looked questioningly at Enver, but didn't say anything.

Opening the brown paper bag, he took a sheep's cheese out and laid it on the table where it became the object of conversation for the next ten minutes. Refusing the glass of Johnnie Walker offered him sheepishly by his son, he then started saying something with more authority in his voice than when he had been speaking about the sheep's cheese.

'Grandfather says Churchill is great man. Very great man,' Spatim translated.

Howard managed to nudge Dan before he pointed out that Churchill was dead.

David wanted to ask if he had ever seen Churchill, but was afraid that it would seem as though he was trying to take the wind out of the old man's sails if he had to say 'no'.

'He fought with Germans during war,' Spatim added. 'Germans and English are both great nations. He would like to go to London one day.'

The old man looked up at them and nodded as Spatim said this.

It occurred to David that he probably spoke English.

At midnight the old man was still holding court, and neither roads nor electricity were referred to again.

By the early hours of the morning the internationals were standing under the light of the porch, watched by the entire family as they put their shoes back on.

As they reached the gates, the door to Balon's hut opened and Balon sloped out.

He pulled the gates back to allow them through, but kept turning his head over his shoulder in the direction of the hut, and forgot to wish them goodnight.

They stepped out into Stengova's main street.

Dan's feet could be heard shuffling through the dust as his body tried to regain its sense of balance after six Johnnie Walkers.

The gates shut behind them.

'Did you hear what the Mayor said about the roads and electricity?' Donatella said. 'He's already tried the same thing with the International Refugee Council when he had them round to dinner.'

'What happened?' David asked.

'They sent him fifty violins. I don't think he was too put out – he knows somewhere along the line he'll get his roads and his electricity.'

She let out a sigh as, tired, her hard-working optimism gave way to the impenetrable chaos that lay at the heart of the matter. 'He's meant to be a very good violinist.'

They didn't say anything after this.

David watched Howard's hand hover over Donatella's back then drop to his side.

Peter started to make off in the opposite direction – back towards the village.

144

'Where are you going?' Howard called after him.

'I'm going looking for a gay bar,' he said, blearily.

'In Stengova? Is there one?'

He shook his head and nearly lost his balance.

'Nothing. D'you know something else? There aren't any veterinary surgeons either. I noticed that. No gay bars and no veterinary surgeons – what does that mean?' He started to walk away.

'We should see him home,' Donatella said.

Howard shrugged. 'Better to let nature take its course.'

They got back to Donatella's and David got into the Fiat and drove slowly out of Stengova, barely able to tell the difference in the dark between fields and road.

When he reached the main road the lorry carrying the prefabricated village he had passed that afternoon was still parked by the toll.

There was no sign of any driver.

Even before he had reached his hut, Balon knew there was something wrong.

He pushed the door open and there was Benny Schmalz, sitting on the single bed pushed up against the far wall. Behind his boots, under the bed, moonlight just reached the row of sheep skulls that he had been collecting over the years. Balon took in the skulls, the bed, the stove, the broom in the corner and the box of woodwork tools, then his eyes went back to Benny Schmalz. He looked at the sheep skulls again. From where Schmalz was sitting he wouldn't know about the skulls. For some reason Balon found this reassuring – even felt that it gave him an ascendancy of sorts.

He didn't say anything; he just stood there waiting for the man to speak.

'So this is where they keep you?' Benny said at last.

Feeling the sudden need to assert himself, Balon said, 'This is my hut.' In the same way he might have said – when in peril – 'My name's Balon.'

Benny nodded in agreement and his smile became – briefly – wider.

Balon ignored this. 'You want to see Enver?' he asked hopefully. Then, remembering, 'Enver's busy tonight.'

'No, I don't want Enver. Enver doesn't look after the old cinema, does he?'

Balon drew his head back slightly.

There was no sense of urgency in Benny, who always managed to get the job done. Part of him was even – much to his surprise – enjoying Balon's open-mouthed company.

'It's you who looks after the old cinema,' he said. 'It's your . . .' he sought around for the right word, looking expectantly at Balon, '. . . kingdom.'

Balon looked unimpressed.

Benny felt himself suddenly bulge with an irritation he had trouble keeping down at Balon's inability – or, worse still, decision – not to join in the game.

'Who was in the old cinema this afternoon? I thought you were the only person who goes in there.'

'And Enver,' Balon said.

'And Enver. But this afternoon there were others. Arsim saw them.'

Benny got up from the bed, the back of his boots rubbing the skulls.

'There are lots of shoes in the old cinema,' Balon said abruptly, hoping to interest Benny Schmalz in this fact and put him off the trail. He didn't want to sacrifice his hoard of shoes but he was willing to if it meant sparing Spatim and Lirije – especially Lirije.

'Shoes?' Schmalz started at this, genuinely taken aback as he realised that the shoes probably meant more to the idiot than the arms stored there. Then, changing tack, he said, 'You're very good at your job, but today you weren't very good. Maybe you shouldn't be doing the job any more.'

Balon stared at his broom – the broom he used to sweep the falling asbestos off the old cinema floor, and his mouth started to work into a wail.

'Nobody's allowed in the old cinema, but this afternoon somebody or some people were there. Who?'

Schmalz wasn't speaking any louder than before, but it felt as though he was yelling.

Balon went over to the stove and picked up a pack of cigarettes. He nervously offered the pack to Benny, who took one and put it in his mouth.

146

After Balon had lit his own, Benny jerked his head as a sign that he was to come over and light his for him.

Balon cupped his hand tenderly over the end of the cigarette in Benny's mouth, protecting it from an imaginary wind. He was at least a foot taller than him.

'You know you're going to have to tell me who was in the cinema, don't you?' Benny whispered through the cigarette.

He suspected more than idiocy from the idiot – just as he suspected more than pain from the wounded or grief from the bereft. He expected more in order to do his worst, and that was his great success in life.

For a while the two men stood in silence, smoking and staring at each other, until they heard the sound of voices outside.

'The gates,' Balon said. 'I need to open the gates.'

Benny followed him, but hung back in the shadows just inside the hut door. He saw Balon look back over his shoulder at him as the internationals filed past into the deserted village street. Through the gates he saw the white light illuminating the northern tip of the camp opposite.

Balon came back to the hut.

The thoughts in his head were straight now – because of the cigarette.

Benny threw his stub down, exhaling and looking to see where it fell on the ground. 'Were any of them at the cinema this afternoon?'

Balon nodded.

Benny Schmalz looked up. 'Which ones?'

Balon went through them in his head. He didn't want to drag the woman into this and the only man he could really remember was the last one who filed past him – Peter Miller. Spatim joked about him, saying he liked boys – especially Albanian boys.

'Only one.'

'Only one of them?'

Balon breathed in deeply. 'The last one – the one who likes Albanian boys.' As soon as he said it, he became convinced of it himself. 'He was at the old cinema this afternoon.'

Benny didn't say anything else, but he did at last move to the door.

Balon thought, for one sickening moment, that he was going to ask him to go with him.

'Not very colourful in here,' Benny said. 'You need more . . . decoration. We should get you some posters.'

Balon was tired; making Lirije and Spatim safe from Schmalz had made him tired. All he wanted was a cup of tea and to smoke another one of his cigarettes.

'You like posters of girls?' Benny asked, showing his teeth.

'I like animals.'

'You like posters of girls with animals?'

Balon looked at him for a moment, almost feeling sorry for him.

'Just pictures of animals – like in the zoo. Monkeys; I like monkeys,' he finished, looking hopefully at Benny Schmalz.

26 ℃

27 May 1999 / Milosević and four other Serbian leaders
are indicted by the UN war crimes tribunal for crimes
against humanity

'You know this man?' Enver said through the handkerchief pressed against his nose, looking down at the body on the bed.

'Of course I know him,' the Australian said, wanting to sit down, but the only place to sit down in the room was on the bed.

The bright sunshine outside only alleviated the darkness in the room slightly. Neither of them thought to open the shutters.

There was a desk with a lamp on it and a dried-flower display. Next to the bed was a cabinet filled with dolls dressed in national costume from all over the world. The sort tourists bought on holiday. Chris Woods found himself crouching down to get a better look. Out of the corner of his eyes he could see Peter Miller's hand lying on the edge of the bed, palm upwards.

'Heroin,' he said, standing up straight again. 'Look at the track-marks on his arms.'

Enver nodded, like he'd guessed as much. 'OD?' he said, liking the sound of the phrase he'd only just recently picked up.

'I guess so.'

'OD,' he said again.

Chris Woods took hold of the corner of the sheet, pulling it back by walking down the length of the bed.

Peter Miller lay uncovered, his head to one side and his mouth open.

Whoever it was who said that dead bodies looked like they

were sleeping, was wrong, Chris thought; dead bodies look dead.

Both men instinctively looked at the dead man's cock, but it didn't mean anything any more. People were 'he' and 'she' – bodies were 'it'.

There was bruising to the wrists and ankles.

Chris knew Peter's history, but didn't want to share it with the Mayor of Stengova.

With a vague sense of hopelessness, he pulled the sheet back over the body as far as the neck – he didn't know what else to do. Then he turned away and walked over to the desk. The sight of adults lying in single beds always depressed him.

Peter Miller's clothes lay in a heap on the floor.

He had always presumed that he was the kind of person who folded them into piles or hung them up neatly in wardrobes or on the backs of chairs.

'I thought you said there were no KLA operatives left in Stengova,' Chris said, turning to the Mayor. 'I've agreed to allow the arms to remain in the old cinema on the condition that no further arms are stored there. That was the first part of our agreement. The second was that all KLA operatives were to be cleared out of Stengova in order not to compromise the daily running of the camp.'

'Why are you talking about operatives? This man committed suicide.' Enver paused, looking angry. 'There are some left, but they don't have business here.'

'So you lied.'

The Mayor shrugged.

'You said all operatives would be cleared out.'

'They don't have business here.'

'But they're still here.'

Enver brought the handkerchief away from his face and put it back into his pocket, drawing out a bag of sunflower seeds instead.

He'd had the same conversation – long distance – with Emshi that morning. And here he was again, being made to feel like a child.

Chris Woods was staring at the watch on the desk, still keeping time, when Arlinda, the woman who owned the house, walked into the room with a piece of paper. She stared at Peter Miller lying on the bed then handed the paper to Chris.

'What's this?' he asked.

The woman turned to Enver, who was starting to eat sunflower seeds from a pile in his hand.

'This is the man's phone bill,' Enver explained. 'He makes lots of international calls. International calls are very expensive.'

'Why's she telling me?'

Enver paused, spitting husks from the seeds into his palm. 'She wants to know – you'll pay?'

'Where's page two of the report?'

The President looked up. 'Page two's on the back of page one,' he said, holding his own copy up.

'You mean you've printed the report out double-sided?'

The President smiled warily. He was afraid of his Finance Minister. He was afraid, in fact, of just about everybody at the moment.

'We're out of paper.'

The Minister shifted his arse around on the chair in an effort to disguise post-lunch flatulence. Then he said, in disbelief, 'Out of paper?'

'Not the whole government, don't worry, just my office.'

The President knew certain things about Goran Brenkov that should have helped him in moments like this. He knew, for instance, that he was embezzling government funds in order to import cartons of miracle hair-gro formula from a supplier in California. He stared at the Finance Minister's head for a while, trying to work out if there was more hair now or not. He was constantly amazed that a man who had lost his faith a long time ago, or possibly never had any, should find it again in a bottle of miracle hair-gro.

'The Prime Minister said there weren't the funds to allocate me a stationery budget.'

He thought about Irina last night, telling him that the difference between a wise man and a clever man was that a wise man sank where a clever man swam. He wasn't exactly swimming right now.

Turning impatiently to the window, he said, 'Can you hear that? Or is it just me?'

They sat and listened. Outside, the low chanting they had been unconsciously aware of for the past ten minutes grew louder. The low, uncertain voices achieved sudden unity and with it increased volume.

'It's the protest rally organised by the National Democratic Party. They're demonstrating against governmental complicity with NATO.'

'Complicity,' the President said, startled. 'We didn't have a choice.'

'There's always a choice – there has to be. There'd be no politics otherwise.'

'I have to see,' the President said decisively, pushing his chair back with difficulty.

The Minister, uninterested, went back to the report in front of him.

In the street below there was a crowd of people with placards. The President watched, for a while, their open-mouthed anger, and read the painted slogans carefully. He was overwhelmed by a sudden rushing envy, wanting to know what it felt like to be down there, to have stayed up late the night before and painted those words. It would be easy, he imagined, to become addicted to such things. No matter what the cause.

'. . . Of course the good side of this is that the refugees will return home,' he heard Goran's voice saying behind him. 'But the down side is that international aid will be pouring into Kosovo and bypass us altogether.' He sighed. 'Apart from the odd orphanage, which will no doubt be inundated with funds and wind up with state-of-the-art computers and battery-operated wheelchairs. They've got this thing about orphans – the internationals – have you noticed?'

The President watched as somebody tried to leave the government building and push his way through the crowd. He thought he recognised his Prime Minister, Luka Mitrovič. Then, the next minute, Luka disappeared. When he reappeared, he was clutching the side of his head and had assumed a more crouching attitude.

The President didn't dislike the idea of Luka being lynched.

A small group of protestors broke away and started to form a circle round him, but just then a wave of police arrived, breaking over the protestors' western flank. Placards started to plummet and the focus of the crowd shifted to the uniformed men among them.

There was no sign of Luka.

'Our GDP's slipped down by 5 per cent since the crisis began, and the number of unemployed is now higher than the number of employed.'

The President turned slowly away from the window to face his Finance Minister.

'Our textiles, metals and chemical industries are dying as we speak.'

The President, smiling, said gently, 'Goran – you really do care.'

The Minister stood up abruptly and the two men stood facing each other in almost identical dark blue, shiny suits, both so badly cut that their hands were forever going to their scrotums to relieve the badly stitched pressure there.

Throwing the report down, Brenkov went to join the President at the window.

Fighting had broken out in the centre of the protestors and individuals were breaking away before being cornered by police.

The President watched a young man in a red T-shirt head off up a blind alley, and instinctively started banging on the window as if it was himself and not the young man he was trying to protect. He could see what was going to happen and was powerless to stop it.

'We're so high up,' the Minister murmured, watching the same thing.

A girl and three boys ran crouching along the wall on the opposite side of the street, finding time to slash the tyres of the OSCE vehicle parked there before disappearing onto the main boulevard where the President could just make out the red glow from the flashing King Burger sign.

His eyes drifted out over the city – which, despite all the movement in the street below, looked still and unaware – to the mountain, Vodna. He picked out the monastery half-way up and the tea hut on top.

'You'll have to go down soon.'

The President felt afraid again. 'Where?'

'Down there.' Goran looked at him, pleased. 'People will expect you to have something to say.'

'But I've got nothing to say.'

The President turned away.

'That's where I proposed to my wife,' he said, his eyes lighting on the mountain once more.

Chris Woods sat tinkering with the executive golf toy on the edge of Irina Yupović's desk, feeling vaguely jealous.

He hadn't imagined her office looking like this, and couldn't think whom she had done business with or what kind of business she had done to be presented with this array of executive gifts.

'Golf?' he said, looking up at her.

She sat back in her chair, impatient. 'The World Bank wants to transform us from a socialist to a market-orientated economy. My executive golf game shows that I'm trying to fulfil their objective.'

'To who?'

'I've got the American Vice-Ambassador's brother-in-law lying in the mortuary at the General, and you're talking about golf.'

He shrugged. 'You were talking about socialism. Which is more relevant?' He paused. 'Which is more irrelevant?'

She said, 'I believe in socialism.' Then leant forward and moved the golf toy out of his reach.

This was the sort of statement he might never have got her to make by probing, yet here she was making it, unprovoked, over a plastic figurine. Letting him view her through a microscope only to suddenly pull away so that even with a telescope – the sort powerful enough to discover new planets with – he wouldn't find her.

'Have you any idea how much this coroner's report is going to cost my department? How much diverting a full-scale enquiry will cost us?'

'Pretty much.' He watched her eyes shifting. 'The Americans might help – it's in their interest. They won't want an enquiry.'

'What, you think I should go to Rudinski – the brother-in-law?'

'They'll want to keep it quiet. It's better for them to have a suicide in the camp than a murder.' He paused. 'Besides, Rudinski's probably met you enough times by now for him to fall in love with you.'

'That might be helpful.'

'Is that how you classify it?'

'Always.'

She lit herself a cigarette.

'Do you want to see the body?' he asked her.

'Why?'

'It might make you less bored.'

'What makes you think I find dead bodies interesting?'

He tried an unsuccessful smile.

'How did he die?' she said.

'Heroin overdose. There was bruising to his neck, wrists and thighs, where I'm guessing he was restrained. His arms were full of old track-marks and whoever did it wanted us to associate the bruising with his sexual practices. It must have been done by someone who either knew him or knew of him. They knew what they wanted us to think.'

What he didn't want to tell her was that Donatella at Women Against War was the one who found him and insisted on sending for a priest so God knows who knew about it now.

She stood up.

'Where are you going?'

'I'm going to see the Americans – I think I'll take John Rudinski out to lunch.'

He watched her check her pocket for her car keys then pick up her mobile and drop it into her bag.

'I keep thinking about what the Mayor said when I was standing over Peter Miller's body in his room in Stengova.'

'What did the Mayor say?'

'He said, "It's three days old."'

'So, what? You want me to feel sad?' she asked, attempting to brush past him, but he stood up suddenly and caught hold of her wrist, squeezing it hard enough to bruise.

She stood staring at him, setting her teeth on edge against the pain. 'I'm surprised by the incident with this American. I believed – when was it? – that you would flush out the operatives in the camp. I believed absolutely, and . . . I was wrong. I don't like being wrong,' she added, jerking her hand suddenly out of his grasp and walking past him through the door.

He called out after her, up the corridor, 'I keep having dreams of us cycling through the streets of Melbourne on a tandem.'

He didn't think she'd respond to that, but she did. 'Dreams of us? There is no us.'

'There could be.'

She stopped walking and turned round to face him. 'Do you know what your problem is? You were read the wrong fairy stories as a child. Didn't your mother ever tell you that the best ones end badly?'

Ellen Rudinski opened her wardrobe to try and find a pair of shoes then saw all her evening dresses hanging up. The sight of so much inactive satin and sequins sent her into hysterics and the cleaner's three-year-old daughter, who found her on all fours in front of the open wardrobe shaking with laughter, burst into tears.

Her mother came running up the stairs.

Ellen tried to sit up and calm down.

'Mrs Rudinski? Something happened?'

She caught her daughter up in her arms.

'I'm fine. It's OK.' She shut the wardrobe door and got unsteadily to her feet.

'We go downstairs now?' the cleaner said, waiting for her.

Ellen nodded and allowed Yasmina to lead her downstairs, sit her at the table and make her herbal tea.

She tried to make amends with the daughter but every time she got close the little girl curled up as far back in the chair as she could.

'Is OK if I smoke?' the mother said.

'Sure. Go ahead.'

Ellen watched her light up. 'Mind if I have one?'

'Please.'

'You have something for the ash?' Yasmina said, looking unsure.

'No, I don't have an ash-tray. I gave up smoking years ago.'

The cleaner looked terrified.

'I'm sorry. But you mustn't.'

'No, I wanted one. Really. It's OK. Calm down — come over here and sit down.'

She felt better once the cleaner, who had been so much in control before, was sitting down at the kitchen table.

'Your daughter — she likes cookies?'

Yasmina whispered something to her daughter, who shook her head and clung to the chair arms.

'She loves them.'

'Great,' Ellen said, suddenly excited.

She got the bag of cookie dough out of the fridge, watched suspiciously by the child.

The child was ugly and spoilt, but she suddenly felt the need to make amends.

The mother finished her cigarette and went over to where the vacuum cleaner was parked.

'No, leave it. Let's all have cookies.'

'But I should finish this first,' Yasmina said, thinking about the five other jobs she had lined up that day.

'Finish it later. Why don't you put some more coffee on – the cookies'll be ready by the time it's done.'

'But your meeting – you'll be late for your meeting – and you mustn't cook in your beautiful suit.'

Ellen started laughing again, and the child shot to the back of her chair. She slid the tray into the oven and ten minutes later put the finished biscuits on to the cooling rack.

The child was still suspicious, but now she smelt chocolate.

'Come and sit down,' Ellen said impatiently to Yasmina, who had got up to fiddle with the vacuum and hadn't made coffee. 'They're best eaten hot.'

She pushed the plate encouragingly towards the child who clung to her mother's arm.

Ellen lit another cigarette, and while she was concentrating on that, the child's hand shot out for the plate, grabbed a cookie and stuffed it in her mouth, her eyes never leaving Ellen.

Yasmina gingerly reached out for one.

'Go on, just eat the damn things,' Ellen urged, suddenly tired by the idea of cookies. The second cigarette had seriously curbed her appetite.

Just then the doorbell went and Yasmina leapt guiltily to her feet.

The child started to whimper.

Yasmina shuffled to the door in her slippers, the child in her arms.

Ellen called out, 'Who is it?'

'Me,' the voice said, sounding British and unsure.

Ellen left the kitchen and went out into the hallway, which was panelled in wood and always felt dark. Through the block of sunshine straight ahead, she made out the British Ambassador's wife.

'That you, Anne?' she said, almost shyly – she'd never called the other woman by her name before.

'I hope so.'

Anne Hargreaves, smiling now, stepped into the hallway and the two women took in each other's suit, made-up face and high heels.

Then, belatedly, Ellen said, 'Come in – come in.'

The cleaner closed the door behind Anne and, her daughter on her hips, made her way thankfully back towards the vacuum.

'Do you know what I was doing?' Anne asked suddenly. 'I was standing by my window, watching your house.'

'You were?'

Anne nodded. 'I was waiting, thinking, if she goes, I'll go.'

'Goes?'

'To International Wives.'

Ellen sighed and turned round. 'You want to come in? I mean, right in? Yasmina,' she called out, 'some more coffee, please.'

They went into the lounge, which, although it was painted in a haphazard series of light blues and greens, came across as grey.

'I was making cookies,' Ellen said.

'Is that your cookie-making suit?'

Ellen sat back in the sofa, trying to work out if she'd ever sat in it before – or the room for that matter. No. Looking around, the room didn't feel familiar.

'I was meant to be going,' she said, 'but I couldn't.'

'Same here,' Anne cut in.

Ellen caught her looking at the toybox down the side of the sofa.

They didn't say anything more until Yasmina entered the room with the coffee, pleased at the sense of formality the visitor had introduced.

'And the toys?' Anne said, wanting their presence in the room to be accounted for.

'Oh – the toys. They're for the kid.'

'The cleaner's child?'

Ellen nodded and took a sip of coffee, watching Anne and trying to hold her cup in the same way. Anne reminded Ellen of her maternal grandmother.

Anne looked down at the box again then at Ellen.

'Toys are horrible things aren't they?'

'Horrible,' Ellen repeated.

The two women smiled at each other.

The cuckoo clock in the hallway started to chime, the mechanism thrusting the wooden bird out into daylight.

Through the wall they heard the sound of the vacuum and, outside the door, the child, who had been watching the cuckoo, run back across the hallway.

Anne Hargreaves said, almost coldly, 'You saw me that day.'

'Yes, you've been haunting me – you know that?' Ellen said after a while. 'The sight of you in that peach kimono.'

'Peach kimono?'

'That's what you were wearing.'

'Was I?'

'Oh, don't forget that – please don't forget it,' Ellen pleaded. 'That kimono – that peach kimono, it almost saved me.'

Then, shaking her head so that the cup rattled in the saucer, 'I thought you had to be dead before you could start haunting people.'

'Oh, I'm not dead,' Anne assured her.

'No, but you're happy, aren't you?'

In the other room, the vacuum cleaner was shut off.

The next minute Yasmina hesitantly appeared at the lounge door.

The child came tottering out from behind her mother, making a beeline for the toybox.

'Lila. No. I'm sorry.'

Ellen stood up. 'It's fine. Leave her.'

She wanted to appear benevolent before Anne Hargreaves.

In the hallway, Ellen counted out the notes, one hand on the latch for the front door. 'Here. Is that right?'

The woman nodded eagerly, pleased.

'Goodbye, Mrs Rudinski. See you next week, Mrs Rudinski. Say goodbye, Lila.'

The child glanced up then quickly hid her face in her mother's jeans.

The woman smiled indulgently and Ellen forced a flicker of affection to cross her face.

'Oh, Mrs Rudinski?'

Ellen, who had been about to shut the door, opened it again. 'What?' she said, impatiently.

'I found a doll under your bed. A very beautiful doll. I put it on the table in the room.'

'Right. Thanks.'

She slammed the door shut.

When she went back into the lounge, Anne, who had got up from the sofa, was standing by the window watching the cleaner and her daughter walking hastily up the drive.

She turned to face Ellen briefly.

'I nearly killed James last night.' She paused. 'And do you know why? Because of the way he was eating. It suddenly struck me as unbearable – absolutely unbearable. I wanted to smash his head on to the table and stick my fork into his neck, all because of the way he was eating. I had to leave the room to stop myself.'

Anne looked out the window again. 'Do you want it?'

'What?'

'The peach kimono.'

'You're leaving?' Ellen asked.

'I might be.'

She sighed, her shoulders lifting up then falling back down again.

'The thing is . . . I wanted to tell you, have been meaning to tell you for some time that it isn't something cheap or quick – it's real. For me it's real.'

Ellen stood watching Anne Hargreaves, trying to keep up with her.

'I wanted to tell you when I saw you that day because I care what you think.'

'Do I think?'

Anne said warmly, 'Oh, you think.'

Ellen considered this. Then suddenly said, 'What's his name?'

'Besim.'

Neither of them moved.

There were no sounds from inside the house and no sounds from outside.

'Thank you,' Ellen said.

Sitting next to Guy in the Women Against War jeep, Aida gave no indication of what she felt on leaving the camp for the first time after how many months? . . . of putting one hundred and ten kilometres between them and Stengova.

When he said, 'Look, the lake,' as they turned a bend in the road and the stretch of water glimpsed through trees opened out below them, she said nothing. It made him want to shout, 'Look. You have to look. If you don't look then you won't see and if you don't see then there's no point to this – to any of this.'

He pressed a button and her window slid down so that she could see more clearly.

After a series of broken glances while trying to navigate the hairpin bends in the single-track road, he realised that what she was actually looking at wasn't the lake, but her reflection in the wing mirror.

When she did turn to him it was to offer him a stick of gum, and he couldn't make out her face because of the sunglasses. Where had the sunglasses come from? Where did the gum come from?

He had wanted to show her something beautiful, and Lake Mavro was meant to be beautiful – *was* beautiful, he thought as the road descended until it was running along the side of the mountains, following the western shore of the lake. To the right the clefts in the mountainside were full of forest and the forest full of wigwam-shaped chalets with rows of logs underneath in the anticipation that the earth would carry on spinning on its axis and the seasons would continue to change.

On the left, overlooking the lake, was a white and blue hotel, whose ugliness – here, where everything had suddenly become so large – didn't amount to much.

Aida had her elbow hanging out the window and her face was now turned towards the lake.

He had pictured her at this moment, smiling – laughing even.

He had pictured a sort of eagerness rising up that would enable them both to take hold of the day and push it towards a point – it didn't matter what point, as long as it was definitive.

He hadn't pictured this silence.

He wanted to be alone with her, but now he just felt lonely.

Things he had planned with such ease lying on the sofa downstairs in the MSF house became, in reality, impossible.

He had contemplated lunch at the Hotel Vista, but when they pulled up in the car park and saw the hoards of UN, OSCE, UNHCR and other 4x4s parked there, he felt her shrink and knew they'd never make it across the threshold into the dining room and sit at a table laid for a five-course lunch. He saw – clearly – that this would be an ordeal and not a pleasure.

So they bought sandwiches from the hut in the car park, where you could hire skis in the winter, and sat on the parapet of a stone bridge, not speaking.

Afterwards, they stood up and brushed the crumbs off themselves, and Guy had to stop himself from saying something when she dropped her half-finished sandwich, still wrapped in clingfilm, on to the bridge and walked away.

The half-eaten sandwich preoccupied him for a good part of the afternoon, and he spent a lot of time working out how to get back to the bridge and dispose of it without her seeing.

They walked to the chairlift that in winter took skiers, and in summer took hunters and walkers, to the top of the mountain, but she simply shook her head at it. Maybe she suffered from vertigo, but there was – at the back of his mind – a nagging suspicion that she was just bored.

He had pictured them strolling along the lakeshore, heavy from lunch, maybe even holding hands. The day would slow right down – they'd slow right down. Instead, here they were straggling along, with Aida drinking loudly from a can of Coca-Cola, still not looking at the view. The empty can ended up – like the sandwich – being dropped on the ground.

The lake couldn't keep them; the mountain couldn't keep them. With nothing to keep them and nothing else to do, they headed back to the car park.

As they got into the jeep a white UN bus pulled up by the kiosk they'd bought their sandwiches from earlier.

Aida watched as a coachload of internationals she didn't recognise, from one of the other camps, piled out – a lot of girls in nothing more than sarongs, bikinis and flipflops – in hot pursuit of rest and relaxation.

It was the first sign of interest she'd shown in anything all day – an acute, unrelenting interest – and Guy didn't put the jeep into gear immediately, letting her get her eyeful.

Eventually she turned away and they drove off back along the single-track road.

'What do they do?' she said suddenly, breaking the almost day-long silence.

'Who?'

'The girls.'

'The girls – they swim.'

'In the lake?'

'In the lake. Then they go to the hotel, shower and change.'

'Change?'

'Put new clothes on.'

Aida nodded, listening intently as if her future depended on it. She turned to him expectantly, wanting more, but not daring to ask.

It touched him; she touched him, in a way he had been waiting to be touched all day.

He smiled at her.

'They go into the restaurant and eat. They start drinking. Some of them don't stop drinking.'

He wished he hadn't said that. She hadn't asked him what he thought; she just wanted to know about the girls in their bikinis. What they did – what they meant.

'They party,' he wound up.

She looked at him, trying to follow the English, trying to work this one out.

Where moments before he had been endeared he suddenly became irritated.

'Party? You know?'

He felt like he was yelling at her, but he wasn't; he was somehow managing to keep his voice steady.

'You can take those off,' he added, lifting his left hand from the steering wheel and pointing to the sunglasses she'd been wearing ever since he met her that morning. 'The sun's gone down – behind the mountains.'

She hesitated then slowly took them off and turned away from him to look out the window.

She didn't ask any more questions.

After lunch, Irina offered to drive Rudinski to the General Hospital, which was situated at the foot of Mount Vodna, on the Medical School campus.

She had taken him to what she called her 'favourite' restaurant for lunch – she hadn't been lying to him. They sat at a table for six, below a moufflon's head mounted on the wall. There was no menu and she had ordered enough dishes for a banquet without consulting him as to his likes and dislikes.

Then, when the young boy who took their order left, blushing, for the kitchen, she had turned to him and said, 'I ordered vege-tarian.'

'How did you know?' he said smiling, polite.

She hadn't said, 'You don't look like a man who eats meat,' like it was a defect, she'd said, 'You look like a man who doesn't eat meat,' like it was a compliment. Then she had told him his brother-in-law, Peter Miller, was dead.

After the meal was over, she'd gone behind the bar herself and pulled up a bottle of the proprietor's home-made raki, pouring them a shot each.

She drank hers standing up with her hand on her hip, then paid the blushing boy.

Rudinski had stood shuffling uneasily outside the restaurant while Irina used the outside loo.

When she joined him, he saw that she had re-applied her make-up.

'We'll take my car.'

Her brutal charm throughout lunch had anticipated his complicity, and here he was, sitting in her car, being driven by her, complicit.

He liked being in her car; he liked the smell of her car. He liked her daughter's paraphernalia in the back, the icon of St George and the Dragon propped up on the dashboard, and the Orthodox cross hanging from the rear-view mirror.

When they reached the hospital she parked behind some pre-fabricated huts that looked like student accommodation. They walked round to the main hospital building, which had once been a private villa, adapted to become an institution.

Once inside, Rudinski, who had a deep, inherent fear of white-tiled walls and shining stone floors, felt nauseous. He followed Irina down the stairwell, walking in the centre and not touching the walls.

'You know where we're going?' he called out as she disappeared round a bend.

Then, when they reached the next bend – how many bends was this now? – 'Where *are* we going?' They seemed a long way underground.

Eventually they reached the bottom, and he managed to catch up with her as they headed down a straight stretch of corridor, passing a room where two women, a blonde and a brunette, were smoking and laughing, their white rubber clogs propped up on a desk. They looked up as he passed, not used to seeing people walking the corridors down here.

The floor was no longer stone, it was lino and smelt of bodies without life. Bodies that no longer had the right to take up space among the living.

The lighting got better and Rudinski made out somebody waiting for them at the end of the corridor – an unimposing man whom he immediately thought of as being dressed as a doctor, rather than actually being a doctor. The man was smiling, like he had good news or was pleased to see them.

They passed through a doorway into the mortuary.

It happened without warning. Rudinski didn't have time to prepare himself, but became immediately conscious of the dead outnumbering the living. For a man who had been shaped by being one of a majority, it was unsettling to find himself suddenly in the minority.

He had been expecting to see only one table and only one body in the room, but instead the room was full of tilted stone slabs with gutters running round the perimeter of them, leading to a larger-scale network of guttering and drainage systems stretching across the entire floor. The guttering hadn't yet been scrubbed, and traces of fluids, in the process of drying, shone. To his left, some woman's hair hung out from under a sheet, over the edge of the table.

There was no sense of urgency.

It reminded him of the orphanage in Colombia he visited, where the thing that had struck him most was that the children weren't waiting for their mothers and fathers to return. If, amid the desolation, corruption and filth, he had found them waiting for that, he might have felt pity, but they weren't. They weren't waiting for anything, and if there was no waiting there were no expectations; if there were no expectations, there was no hope. This is what the mortuary reminded him of – orderly rows of disorderly bodies with no sense of life; of ever having been alive.

'He is here, isn't he?' Irina said at last, turning, irritated, to the doctor who had followed them in.

The man smiled and gestured at Rudinski, as if he should lead the way.

Rudinski looked down to make sure that he wasn't about to step into a gutter or already standing in one.

The doctor stepped towards a stone table just off-centre. Rudinski anxiously followed and watched him pull back the stained green cloth covering Peter.

Irina seemed to have receded, and now things felt sticky round the edges in a way they hadn't done at lunch-time. Like they might attract flies.

He looked at Peter's face, and for the first time in his life felt like touching his brother-in-law. Peter's right eye, which had drooped ever since his run-in with the Kenyan police – a reason he could never bear to look at him – had, now it was shut, regained its symmetry with the left eye.

Irina came over to stand beside him, more out of a sense of thoroughness than curiosity. She needed this business to be water-tight; she needed the man standing in the room with them – the 'doctor' – to stop smiling. It showed a level of involvement that wasn't required of him. This was the sort of man you hoped never to have to need – the sort of man you always did end up needing, one way or another.

Rudinski stared; he got his eyeful of a man he had never loved; a man he had, for as long as he remembered, disliked. Then his hand went out instinctively for the cover, suddenly embarrassed that Peter was naked when he'd had no choice in the matter.

'Is this Peter Miller?' Irina said, looking at the dead man then Rudinski.

Angry, Rudinski said, 'Who the hell d'you think it is?'

'There's meant to be bruising to the neck, wrists and thighs – it's not so clearly defined,' she said to the doctor.

'The body's decomposing as we speak – and was already in an advanced stage of decomposition when it was found this morning. The heat . . .'

'Yes, the heat.'

'When did he die?' Rudinski said suddenly, looking at both of them.

Irina turned to the doctor.

'Three days ago,' he said, still smiling. 'We estimate time of death to be around 3.00 a.m. on May 24th.'

'He's been dead three days?' Rudinski said, to Irina this time. 'Nobody noticed? Nobody missed him?'

'Have you got the papers?' she said to the doctor, ignoring Rudinski.

He nodded and took her over to a desk against the wall, near the doorway.

She studied them by the light of the desk-lamp.

There was the sound of voices in the corridor, laughing voices coming closer, and Rudinski thought of the two laughing nurses he had seen earlier.

Irina's head flicked up, listening.

The doctor went to the doorway.

Irina remained poised, standing over the desk as the voices got closer. Then a door opened, the voices receded, a door closed, and the voices vanished.

She remained motionless for a further five seconds, then went back to reading the document in front of her.

Rudinski covered Peter Miller up and walked carefully over to the desk.

'I think I was the last person he spoke to,' he said quietly, to Irina Yupović's back.

'What did he say?' she said sharply, turning round.

'He wanted to speak to Ellen.' He whispered his wife's name. 'I wouldn't let him.'

She stared at him a moment longer then held out the documents. 'You can read these and sign them or just sign them.'

'What are they?'

'Cremation certificate. Don't look at me like that. We discussed this over lunch.'

'You went to Branko's?' the doctor by the doorway cut in. 'For lunch?'

Irina ignored him.

'Branko's – the best raki in the Republic,' he said, turning to Rudinski.

'It's eight pages long,' Rudinski said, flicking through the document. 'What is this?'

'I'm a bureaucrat, Mr Rudinski. I like long documents – I like rubber stamps. I like things to look official.'

'But whose signatures are these? How long ago was the document drawn up?'

'I wasn't notified of your brother-in-law's death until this morning – these were drawn up shortly afterwards. We have to move quickly and quietly. Cremation is the most efficient means of disposing of the body. Cremation is . . . necessary.' She tried to smile but couldn't. Then added, 'I'd like to be cremated.'

Rudinski stared at her. 'You would?'

He signed the documents. He didn't know what else to do.

Irina put her briefcase on the desk and the documents inside.

Then she walked back over to where Peter Miller lay and, bending over him, pulled the cover back.

'Your wife – she looks like him?' Rudinski stayed where he was. 'Yes,' he said. 'Yes, she does.'

★

167

Rudinski opened the front door and screwed his face up at the music he heard playing on the stereo. Even though the sun had long since gone down, there were no lights on inside. He walked through the dark house to the kitchen at the back, where he stood by the French windows looking out into the garden.

After a while he made her out, lying on the sun lounger, her hair poking through the slats. He saw her hand stretching down for the glass then knocking it over. She swung her legs round so that she was sitting up. The next minute she had the bottle in her hand.

Then she looked up, straight at him.

He didn't know whether she could see him or not, but they stayed like that for a good sixty seconds.

The bottle must have been empty because she dropped it on to the lawn, swung her legs back on to the lounger and lay down again. She wasn't wearing shoes.

Rudinski sighed, walked over to the fridge, and opened it. The light from inside temporarily illuminated the kitchen table where there was a plate with a cookie on it. Ellen hadn't baked cookies in how long? He wondered what the occasion had been. The lone cookie struck him as somehow ominous, like it had been saved for someone special. He turned his back on it and made himself a gin and tonic.

He had got used to the taste two years back, but still wasn't convinced he really liked the drink. But then doing things he didn't like was more in his nature than doing things he liked. His mother had prepared him – fanatically – for all the sacrifices he would have to make in life, but for none of the joys. She had said, when he announced his plan to marry Ellen Miller, that he would have his work cut out for him. She'd shaken her head, sighed, and given the dog lying on the sofa next to her some harsh strokes, but he could see that she was pleased. Pleased that his choice would bind him. She had a fear of freedom, and hadn't raised her children so much as trained them. Now his two daughters were passing through her hands. She spoke on the phone as if they were her own. He spoke to her on the phone – from the embassy – as if they were her own. Ellen didn't come into it for either of them. If people were broken, his mother tended to leave them that way. If they weren't, she chipped at them until the cracks started to appear.

He shut the fridge door and took a sip of his gin and tonic, his eyes now accustomed to the semi-dark as he walked over to the hi-fi system.

The man singing got round to telling him 'Lulu's back in town', before he cut him out. It was bad enough Ellen listening to that stuff, but when it played to itself it was even worse.

He went back to the French windows, opening one of the doors and stepping out into the garden.

Ellen must have heard the door opening and his footsteps, but she didn't turn round.

He stood just behind the lounger, looking down at the crown of her head then out at the city. Cities tended to lose their nationality at night when the electricity was switched on, and this one was no exception. He liked being up high. He felt safe up here and had liked the house on the hillside as soon as he saw it. Had he also thought that up here on the hillside they might somehow get things back together even if only enough to make amends to each other? Yes – briefly.

He realised that his hand was nearly touching his wife's black hair. This must have happened unconsciously, and he moved away to sit down at the table they hadn't yet eaten a meal at. There were about two metres of lawn between them now.

Ellen still hadn't turned to look at him or acknowledge his presence in any way.

'What's that you're wearing?' he said.

'It's a peach kimono.'

'Haven't seen it before – did I buy you that?'

'No, you didn't buy it me.'

After a while, he said, 'Can you hear that?'

'What?' She turned to face him at last.

They listened as the breeze brought the sound of a voice to them, singing unaccompanied.

'Oh, that,' she said. 'He's been at it for hours – poor guy must be nearly hoarse.'

Rudinski screwed his head round, trying to find the summit of the mountain against the night sky.

'It's coming from up there.'

'The monastery,' she reminded him.

'Of course, the monastery,' he said, reassured by this.

The breeze brought the voice round again, then the lounger creaked as Ellen shifted her weight.

'I saw some of them monks once.'

'You did?' he said, not believing her.

'That day I tried to climb the mountain. I saw three of them and couldn't believe how miserable they looked. For being so holy and all, I mean. I sensed a great . . .' she carried on, less sure of herself, '. . . evil in them.'

'Evil?'

'I don't know – like there was a lot they needed to ask for-giveness for.'

'But they were monks.'

'You're so damned stupid sometimes, John,' she muttered quietly.

A helicopter flew low overhead.

'You cold?' he asked.

His sudden attentiveness made her laugh. 'No, I'm not cold.'

He watched her crane her neck up at the helicopter and started to rub his hand along his left leg. He thought about Peter laid out in the mortuary that afternoon, and the three days it had taken for anyone to realise he was missing.

Peter had rung the house four days ago – that must have been the day before he died – wanting to speak to Ellen. Rudinski had told him that his sister had popped so much Valium she was in a coma, then hung up.

'Ellen,' he said softly, watching her get up and accidentally kick the empty wine bottle so that it rolled across the lawn until it banged against the legs of the chair he was sitting on.

She picked up her shoes and started walking across the lawn towards the house. She looked good in the kimono – here in the garden, at night. No, he definitely hadn't bought it.

'Where are you going?'

She had one hand on the door – the other covering her mouth as she yawned. 'To bed. I've got an early flight tomorrow morning.'

Rudinski stood up.

'Early flight where?'

She didn't answer.

'Were you thinking of telling anybody?'

'I don't have anybody to tell.'

She yawned again, not bothering to put her hand over her mouth this time.

'You know what I've been thinking – these last few weeks – I've been thinking how I always thought it was better to take things for granted – even become bored of them – than to know how they worked. How they really worked. 'Cause that would mean being amazed and having your credulity stretched. And now . . .'

'You won't go,' he cut in.

'I'll go – I'm going.'

'What about Peter?'

'I love Peter,' she said. 'But he doesn't need me.'

She dropped her shoes on to the patio and slipped her feet into them. Her hand looked white, gripping on to the doorframe.

For a moment he thought she knew that Peter was dead – she suddenly seemed capable of anything.

'How did we get here?' he asked.

'That's not fair,' she said, raising her voice for the first time that evening. 'That was meant to be my question. I've been waiting to ask that question for twenty years.' There was genuine outrage in her voice, as if he'd stolen the last thing from her it was possible for him to steal. This was meant to be her question; the one that came storming out from behind the bottles of wine and boxes of Valium; from under her daughters' beds in their dormitories at Wellington. The question that had as good as replaced her spine over the years.

'That was my question,' she said again, then disappeared into the kitchen, leaving the door open, and was soon lost in the darkness.

Rudinski was left in the garden, staring up at the house, watching lights go on and off as she made her way between bathroom and bedroom.

Then the lights went out.

29°c

9 June 1999 / NATO Secretary General calls for a suspension of NATO bombing after evidence that Serb forces are withdrawing from northern Kosovo – UN Resolution 1244 adopted, setting up UN Interim Administration in Kosovo

A kilometre away, the twin spires of Stengova's mosque shifted in the afternoon heat. Blinded by sweat, David nearly sent a man, his wife and their donkey into the ditch, only just managing to miss them by taking a short cut through a field of what would become sunflowers.

When he reached the village, he parked the car and headed straight for the community centre that Donatella was trying to get finished in time for the speeches that would be made there prior to the party that evening. Colin Roberts from UNICEF, Des Mortimer from World Food Programme (who had done something unspeakable in Ethiopia, and had recently been promoted to Head of Mission in Kosovo in order to dispel rumours), and Heike Schiff from OSCE – among other high-profile humanitarians – had all been sent invitations, but had not yet committed themselves. Under the weight of their half-promises, Donatella was running around screaming out dimensions to the rug dealer standing smoking at the top of the stairs. Who, showing no apparent sign of excitement at the large order being placed and the premium price agreed, turned to go.

'I know you can't make any promises,' she called out to his receding back, 'but please try and get the rugs here by tonight. Just try.'

There was a roof on the upper storey now, but still no walls. In the empty space where there should have been concrete there was a clear view of the mosque, and sky.

David and Donatella stood at the edge of the floor and watched the man start to get into his van then, recognising someone, get back out and walk towards the pizza parlour.

She started to chew on her nails, staring at some fixed point on the horizon where a rug dealer was doing battle with UN officials.

'I heard about Peter Miller,' David said.

'You did? I'd ask you how, but I haven't got the energy. It was a heroin overdose,' she added.

'That's what I heard.'

'That's what I was *told*,' she said.

'What happened?'

'I don't know.'

'You don't know or you don't want to know?'

She sighed, at last turning to look at him, a smudge of dirt across the bridge of her nose. 'For once – I don't want to know. It's over.'

She had something else to say and he waited to hear it.

'I sent for the priest.'

'I thought he was meant to be dead when they found him.'

'He was, but I still sent in the priest.'

David nodded. 'That's what I heard as well.' He paused. 'Did it cost you?'

'It cost me. Where's Howard?' she said suddenly.

'I'll find him for you.'

She nodded then turned away.

In the downstairs room where a prayer meeting had been held the day he was first shown the building, Genevieve from repro-ductive health was sticking Polaroids of mothers and children on to a piece of card. Next to her, Nadia was making photomontages of children she had worked with, all smiling. Her now-infamous production of *Little Red Riding Hood* was being staged that evening, after the speeches.

David walked back through the village to the camp and found Howard down at the circus tent – erected that morning – with the German technicians, who had enough sound and lighting equip-ment to hold a concert in a stadium. They had arrived at dawn with the sun and the heat and been working incessantly ever since.

Howard turned round as David tapped him on the shoulder.

'Ah, the journalist.'

'Donatella needs you,' David said, ignoring the jibe.

'Where is she?'

'Up at the centre.'

Howard started to walk away, then stopped.

'"Needs" me? Are you sure?'

David nodded, watching him. 'I'm sure.'

Howard disappeared without another word.

One of the technicians jumped off the stage, a blood-soaked handkerchief round his fist.

'Big party tonight,' the German said breathlessly, 'big music, big dancing.'

'That's right,' David agreed, his eyes on the other man's fist.

He hadn't decided whether he was staying for the party or not. Somehow he couldn't picture himself dancing.

The evening was due to start at 7.00 p.m., but by 5.00 p.m. the lack of metropolitan nightlife was finally taking its toll on Nadia and Giulietta, crammed into $3m^2$ worth of newly tiled bathroom in the Women Against War house.

Usually, during daylight hours they were able to talk semi-coherently about the suffering of innocents and the lack of tarmac in Albania. Now, however, inebriated with anticipation they were alternately laughing and crying as they jostled for mirror space.

'I've never seen you in blue before,' Giulietta said, her elbow wedged between her colleague's breasts.

'Spatim says it's his favourite colour.'

'I prefer you in black.'

Nadia managed to shrug despite being in the middle of applying copious amounts of mascara.

'I heard that Dan Hale's sleeping with another woman,' she said.

'What – Olive?'

'No – a Swede.'

This cut to the quick, as anticipated.

'You've seen her?'

'Heard of her. She's a financier for World Food Programme . . . a blonde financier for World Food Programme.'

'Well, I heard that Spatim's getting married,' Giulietta said, regaining her balance, as Nadia staggered into the toilet cistern.

'Who to?'

'The Mayor's daughter.'

'Never seen her.'

'No one has. But she does exist.'

'Arranged marriages also exist.'

'From what I heard,' Giulietta said, drawing a thin brush along her lower lip, 'this isn't arranged – far from it. From what I heard . . .'

'You already said that,' Nadia cut in.

'From what I heard,' Giulietta persisted, 'it's true love.'

'How long have you known this?' Nadia demanded.

Giulietta shrugged.

Nadia spent another minute trying to touch up her lipstick then broke down in tears. 'Don't tell me you're not so lonely sometimes you could just . . . just,' she said through tears of molten foundation.

Giulietta, overwhelmed, broke down as well and took Nadia in her arms.

Fifteen minutes later they were dabbing at each other's faces and rapidly re-applying their make-up.

David sat at the end of the back row, looking out through what should have been a wall, at the stars. There were two banks of chairs – all full – facing the Mayor of Stengova and other local dignitaries, who, unannounced, had arrived in the back of the minibus wearing matching long dark coats, despite the temperature. They flanked Enver on either side, and the two mayoral eagles – hoisted up by a pulley from the road below – were rearing their heads above his shoulders.

The rug, which had arrived too late, was rolled up behind them, but the electricity worked and the bare bulbs hanging from the drying cement ceiling would soon make the upper storey of the community centre, and all those sat in it, visible for miles around.

Donatella stood in front of the local barons with Spatim, who was wearing a new Evil Dead T-shirt for the occasion. Speaking in her heavy English accent, she paused every now and then for him to translate. Against the feudal backdrop of the Mayor and his colleagues she looked frail, and her carefully planned, heartfelt speech did the best it could to withstand translation.

All the internationals from the camp were there, as well as most of the male population of the village over the age of eighteen. Colin Roberts and an associate from UNICEF had turned up an hour ago, and OSCE had in the end sent Charles Winnerton, an older and more important version of Heike Schiff.

Des Mortimer had looked at the gaping absence of walls with condescension when he first arrived, but now felt that the view of the mosque to his left lent the evening a certain substance and weight. So much so that, when Donatella finished speaking, he was the first to start clapping.

Before the sound of clapping died down, Enver stood up and began his speech, having to raise his voice above the unrepressed screams coming from downstairs where twenty under-eights were waiting to come up and perform *Little Red Riding Hood*.

There was, if anything, more at stake for Enver this evening than there was for Donatella, but his speech – unlike hers – was effusively insincere. Unable to display his full power and make the internationals fear him, he was exercising the only other option available in the circumstances: imploring them to distrust him. Nobody had expected anything less, and by the time the interminable speeches came to an end and the screaming children ran up the stairs and down the aisle towards the front of the room, everybody genuinely believed that they were striving to make the world a better place.

Enver sat back down, gathering the ends of his coat up and mumbling something to Spatim, who sat down next to him.

The children stood giggling in front of them, cardboard masks awry – waiting for Nadia, who was trying to erect the cardboard cottage, to tell them to begin.

Nadia was too highly strung to right the lopsided cottage and ordered the children to the side of the impromptu stage, unconcerned by the absence of walls separating them from the night outside, or the shriek as the wolf lost his footing near the edge of the floor.

'The children', she said, turning to face the audience, 'are now going to perform *Little Red Riding Hood* for you.'

She started to clap and the audience of internationals joined in loudly.

They had heard countless similar announcements in countless

176

other halls across the world. Some of them were even unwittingly looking for their own children behind the masks.

The faces of Enver and his entourage were unmoved, and none of them clapped.

Little Red Riding Hood progressed beyond the reaches of stage management. Children walked into cardboard trees, the cottage toppled, the wolf kept taking his mask on and off, and Little Red Riding Hood refused to speak.

The internationals loved it; the applause was riotous.

Nadia, getting up to take her bow among the debris of masks and costumes, was close to tears.

The children, who were so high by now that they had to be scraped off the ceiling, were taken back to the camp.

David followed the internationals out of the community centre towards Petri's restaurant, where a reception had been organised before the party started in the circus tent.

The lighting inside Petri's was low.

The Mayor and his barons, still in their coats, sat at the table on the balcony talking among themselves and were soon forgotten by the internationals, now obsessed with seating plans. Only the elderly VIP from OSCE, Charles Winnerton, was seen briefly at the Mayor's table – during which time Enver managed to negotiate a four-wheel drive for Stengova out of him. In order, he explained, to get food to outlying villages on roads that were impassable during the winter.

Later the Mayor loudly and publicly thanked Charles Winnerton for his generous gift to the people of Stengova, and pledged to name the four-wheel drive Charlie, after its donor.

The steak was thin and overcooked, and David couldn't help thinking of the cow he had seen strung up from the lamppost on his first day in Stengova. Most people were too drunk by this stage to care. The Bulgarian waitresses, slouching between the kitchens and restaurant, had the bodies of whores and faces of executioners, offering prospects with alarming potential to all but the most far gone.

A band quietly installed itself and a couple of loudspeakers to the left of the bar. Enver, although pleased at the outcome of the four-wheel drive discussion, was preoccupied by thoughts of the singer – Lori – soon to perform, and for whom he still had a childish fascination. In his upstairs office he had lids from chocolate boxes with her picture on stuck to the wall. He sat back in his seat and waited, watching one of the waitresses who had been in the minibus the day he brought Sylvie across the border – Sylvie, who had sat on the end of the bed that morning in the dressing gown he bought her – with birds and flowers embroidered all over it – wishing she could just sit there in an old cardigan and slippers because she was feeling homesick, but was too proud to say.

The lighting, which had been gradually dimming all evening, was now just a dull glow.

When the band started up they were loud, and the internationals turned expectantly towards the source of the music.

A microphone crackled, and something silver shivered at the back of the restaurant.

From where he was sitting, David could see the silver. Then there was gold, of sorts, as light fell on to Lori's blonde hair. That night it was enough for everyone, and when the singing started they all began to clap and cheer.

The first song finished and another one started, but people soon lost track as one song ran into another.

Lori, whose credentials lay in a long genealogy of singers, but who had little talent, made her way professionally from table to table – every now and then letting her arm pass along the back of an international male. Cameras emerged and photographs were taken. At some point, people got up and started to dance. Even Des Mortimer from World Food Programme, with an excited laugh, got to his feet.

At a nod from Enver, somebody threw Lori a white handkerchief and she used it to lead the internationals, Albanian-style, in a traditional dance. For a while, as they came together in a circle, they tried to follow. Then the circle broke into a line and people started to improvise, dragging up memories of half-learnt steps from nights spent in Greek tavernas long ago. Lori laughingly went along with it for a while and Enver's table even tried clapping, in an attempt to keep chaos at bay.

Guy, seeing David, broke away from one of the shuffling groups of dancers and dropped down on to the banquette opposite him.

'I didn't notice you earlier,' David said.

Guy wiped his face with his shirt sleeve. 'When did we last see each other? Mid-May sometime?'

'I've been in Stengova before now – asking after you.'

'You have?'

'I was told you've found a girl.'

'A girl . . .' Guy started, then broke off, mumbling rapidly, 'I need some help.'

'Money?'

He shook his head. 'Advice.'

'I'm drunk,' David said.

Guy kept looking steadily at him.

'About what?' David said, relenting.

'Visas.'

Lori was leading the chain of dancers up the steps, round the back of the restaurant and towards their table. Looking round, David realised that they were the only ones not dancing. Every now and then someone would fall into a table or over a chair and the line would discard them, barely giving them time to crawl away before being trampled over.

'What makes you think I know anything about visas?'

'When you first got here you went to see someone in the visa department at the American embassy, and you've got a friend who's an MP,' Guy hissed triumphantly. 'I looked through your diary on the plane.'

David felt as though he had been talking in his sleep. 'That amounts to nothing. There are no strings in that lot worth pulling.'

He leant forward unsteadily.

Guy's face looked fresher than ever, but the eyes were blood-shot.

Lori paused briefly at their table. Up close, David recognised her face from the chocolate boxes in the supermarket. Closer still, as she beckoned him to join the dance, he saw silver sequins covering unhealthy flesh, a heavily made-up face and, when she opened her mouth to smile, grey rotting stumps where teeth should have been. Then she veered away.

'You do know people, don't you?' Guy insisted after a moment's silence.

'Of course I know people. It's one of the prerogatives of growing old,' he said, determined once more not to be moved by the young man's naïve belief in him.

The fact that Guy had chosen personal happiness above personal gain was about as much of a change as his system could cope with. He wasn't about to save the world but he had taken measures to save himself, which meant that he wasn't about to aid in its destruction either. He had come through cynicism and out the other side.

'Christ, there'll be someone here in the camp, churning out visas by the hour at a cost – ask any of the refugees. The last thing you need to do is go through diplomatic channels.' He finished the bottle of beer in front of him. 'What's her name?'

Guy looked away.

'Where are you planning on taking her?' Guy, who had been watching the dancers, turned to stare at David. 'You don't know, do you – hadn't thought of that? Take her somewhere nice – take her to Monte Carlo, for Christ's sake.'

The thought of Monte Carlo flitted briefly across Guy's mind, but he pushed it away, along with memories of alcoholic sweats and sales of £1 million plus second homes . . . his mother's pride in him, which had increased in direct proportion to his self-disgust . . . her own alcoholism . . . and her carefully concealed misanthropy, which made even her love for him conditional.

He pushed his chair back and without another word disappeared among the dancers.

'Whatever you do, don't ever hate her if she turns out to have an appetite for all the things you've renounced in life,' David called out after him, but he was gone.

The sound of the dancers shrieking got louder and louder until at some point, nobody could remember when exactly, Lori passed the white handkerchief to Colin Roberts, who reluctantly relinquished his sweaty grip on her. He was the only one to notice her going.

Enver's table had long since emptied and he and Spatim were waiting for Lori outside the back of the restaurant where her Mercedes was parked. It took some time for the band to realise that – apart from the dancers – they were no longer accompanying anyone. One by one they faltered, cautiously packing their instruments away, and leaving quietly as Lori had done earlier, by the back door. Not that anybody noticed their departure.

The internationals had subconsciously started singing themselves, and where before they had been trying to follow an intricate pattern of seemingly simple steps, they were now just stamping. Lori's strange cadences, neither fully eastern nor fully western, had been replaced by a robust chant.

David saw that the Mayor and his barons had left, and then wondered whether this wasn't part of some plan. Whether masked gunmen weren't, after all, about to come crashing through the glass-fronted restaurant and start open firing.

He stifled his growing panic by pouring a glass of vodka from the bottle somebody had opened and left on the table. Afterwards, he pushed the bottle covetously between his legs. There was now a constant banging inside his head and he knew he needed water. He became aware that he was no longer sitting up straight; he had fallen over to the side, his head pressed against the wall. With an effort he managed to sit upright again.

The dancers had left the restaurant.

Through the windows, Colin Roberts, still in the lead, was clearly visible pulling the long line of internationals across the pavement. They no longer looked like they were dancing, but cavorting instead as they crossed the dust-ridden main street and headed off towards the camp's perimeter fence. On cue, an almighty stereophonic boom rose up from the circus tent as a signal from the Germans that the party was ready to start.

The door shut on the last international. A plate knocked by somebody's arm came spinning to a halt; a wavering chair toppled over with a suit jacket still hung on the back of it, and a faint odour of hash hung in the air. In the restaurant's sudden silence he felt the urge – the first real urge – to write.

Petri emerged from the kitchen and a couple of the Bulgarian waitresses materialised once more and started clearing the tables. Earlier in the evening, David had half-contemplated one of them because she reminded him of a girlfriend he once had in Valencia. At last he managed to get her attention and she walked begrudgingly over with a pile of dirty plates stacked in her arms.

'Excuse me, do you have any paper?' David managed to get out.

'What do you mean "paper"?' she said, immediately suspicious rather than pleased to find that he spoke a variant of her mother tongue.

'Just paper.'

'What paper? Like bill? Everything's free tonight,' she said with disgust.

'No, just paper.'

'What's "just paper"?'

'Something to write on.'

'Write what?'

David stared at her for a moment. 'Does it matter?'

He wondered whether she had – at some stage in her life – been trained to hold interrogations instead of conversations, and was about to give up when her face, suddenly and unbelievably, broke into a smile.

'You want to write something to me?'

Before he had time to answer, she said, 'I'll get you something,' and walked off with the stack of plates. She soon returned and put three napkins on the table in front of David.

'Thanks. Thanks very much.'

She watched him unfold the first napkin and spread it straight, but after a few more minutes shook her head and went back to cleaning tables.

He had just finished filling the first napkin when the door suddenly opened and Marcus, the MSF doctor, tired after having just finished his shift in the medical tent, walked into the restaurant in search of food.

The Norwegian sniffed the air as though he could smell the internationals' hysteria and Lori's silver sequins.

'Can I get anything?' he called out.

'Big party here tonight,' Petri shouted from the back of the restaurant.

'I know.' The Norwegian yawned and sat down near David. 'Where did everybody go?'

'Out there somewhere,' David said, pointing vaguely into the night. 'They were dancing.'

'Dancing?'

'They're having a party in the tent.'

Marcus lit a cigarette. 'And you're not going to the party?'

David shook his head. 'I don't dance. I don't . . .' He lost his drift.

He could barely hold the bottle steady enough to get the vodka into the glass. In fact, his lap was wet, he noticed, as liquid trickled over the side of the table. Cursing, he used the napkin he had written over to wipe himself.

Marcus was about to say something when a Bulgarian waitress appeared with the remains of an earlier meal, hastily reheated.

Petri shrugged an apology and placed it on the table himself.

The Norwegian was beyond caring, ate rapidly, and pushed his empty plate to one side.

Then he remembered David, slumped in the corner.

'You OK?' he called over.

David gurgled, but didn't manage to speak.

'Is he OK?' Marcus asked Petri.

Petri affected concern.

'Hey – you OK?' Marcus called again.

David pawed at the table, trying to sit up straight.

'What is he?' Marcus asked.

'English, I think,' Petri answered.

Marcus stood up, weary but determined, and walked over to where David was sitting.

'Can you stand up?' he said to him.

David held his arms up in front of him, like a child waiting to be picked up, and Marcus dragged him out of the seat.

David wavered, his back bent over, looking as though he was about to drop on to all fours then Marcus led him over to the other table and made him sit down.

'I don't think anything's the matter with him,' Marcus pronounced at last. 'Apart from alcohol.'

Petri didn't care; he just wanted them gone.

'Look, I'll take him home with me tonight,' the Norwegian said, hoisting David up so that he was bearing nearly all the other man's weight.

Petri smiled encouragingly and saw them out into the night, full of the repetitive boom of the party coming from inside the camp.

Marcus steered David up the street past the mosque and community centre towards the MSF house.

He put David into Guy's room. Guy was out at the party and unlikely to return home that night. Pushing David into the bed, he then went downstairs and came back up with a jug of water, which he failed to get him to drink.

David tried to remember what country he was in, but his head was spilling over.

Two minutes later, before working out where in the world he was, he fell asleep.

★

The sky was dark now, but it was still warm. There were enough leaves on the vines to be moved by the breeze and the sound of them made the night seem warmer still. The grapes would be good this year, the President thought looking around him.

From an open upstairs window, he could hear repetitive electronic music coming from the Playstation game Elena and a friend from school were playing, but tonight this didn't bother him.

He felt an acute, piercing happiness and looked across the table at his wife, who was frowning.

'They've already started taking arms across from Kukes in Albania to Prizren,' she said slowly, thinking as she spoke. 'Anything they've got in Stengova will disappear over the border in the next couple of days.'

'Let it go,' he said.

'Let it go? Why?'

He leant forward and poured them both a glass of wine; the empty plates from dinner rattling as his knee jogged the table.

'We know the arms are there – I've got to *do* something with that knowledge,' Irina persisted.

He sighed, tired of the talk; tired of waiting for her to let go of the day.

'What does your Australian say?'

'He doesn't say anything – he's gone silent on me. I think he's been negotiating with his Albanian Mayor and cut a better deal for his organisation with him. The Mayor probably gets to keep the arms and in return the camp becomes KLA-free, which means that Chris Woods gets an easy life and we get neither arms nor operatives.'

'Maybe. Alternatively, he could just be letting it go.'

Irina looked at him, preoccupied, and pulled the glass of wine towards her. Then unexpectedly added, 'You sound exhausted.'

'I am. It comes from running all the time just to stand still.'

'I've never tried that.'

'You don't have to – you just stand still and glide forward. I've never worked out how.'

'Does that make me lucky or unlucky?'

He shook his head.

'Lucky, I guess.'

'I saw an unlucky man the other day – lying in the mortuary at the General.'

The President stared at his wife. Her eyes were watering. In most people that was a sign of the onset of tears, but he didn't think he'd ever seen her cry before. He sat back in his chair, one short leg crossed over the other, wondering what on earth he was going to do if she started crying. It was always him who cried – never her.

'The CIA – the fucking Albanians – us . . . we all thought he was into the heavy stuff: arms, drugs. We all thought he was somebody, and because of that, he's dead. But he wasn't, he was nobody. You know what that means? Being nobody means you're innocent.'

He leant forwards and put his wine glass on the table.

'If he got caught up in things then he was just stupid.'

She shook her head. 'He wasn't stupid, he was innocent – I told you that.'

Her eyes were definitely shining now.

'I had a vision, Orgi. The American was standing there looking at his brother-in-law, and I went over to stand next to him, but d'you know what I saw when I looked down? I saw a ten-year-old child lying there. The Vice-Ambassador's brother-in-law was thirty-eight years old, and I saw a ten-year-old boy. I had a vision right there, standing in the mortuary,' she said, raising her voice now. 'I could hear the American talking to me, not a word of it going in, and the only thing I could do to keep myself together was ignore him and ask for the cremation papers. I didn't read them.'

'Sometimes . . .'

'No,' she said, violently. 'Don't explain it to me.'

'You're tired,' the President said.

'I don't get tired.'

'That's right – I forgot.' He paused. 'You want to go away?'

'Where?'

'I don't know where – somewhere – we could grow our own vegetables – have another six kids.'

He sat forward, his hands gripping the chair arms, his belly creeping along his thighs.

'It's what most people want,' he said, offended by her silence. 'To be able to live their lives in peace.'

'That doesn't sound unreasonable, Orgi, but we're hardly at war here.'

'And we're not at peace.'

He looked up through the vine leaves. The electronic music had cut out and he could hear Elena and her friend, laughing. He heard Elena's laughter above the other girl's – not because it was louder, but because he knew it; knew the sound of it.

'My mother used to say that a successful man is one who's shaken so many hands, he's lost the lines in his palms. I don't know if I want to be that man – that kind of man.'

Irina, whose head had also looked up at the sound of her daughter's laughter, turned to face him.

'So what are you trying to say – you wish you'd never grown up?'

'No, not that, it's just sometimes I can't quite see the point. Where's being grown up got us?'

He looked across the table at her.

She said, 'It's not all bad.'

She didn't raise her eyebrows as she said it; it was more like her face uncrossed itself. She did that sometimes – uncrossed her face in the way some women uncrossed their legs.

She did it at functions when they were standing on opposite sides of the room. Their eyes would meet and it was like she was standing right in front of him, their noses pressing up against each other.

'I believe you, Orgi,' she was saying. 'I believe in you.'

Aida watched her father knocking on the door to the MSF house, which had frosted glass.

The porch light, shining down on them, was making him nervous.

She stared at the bandage wrapped around her arm that had been soaked in cow's blood – a precautionary measure to get them out of the camp that, in the event, hadn't been necessary because of the chaos caused by the party.

They could hear the boom and the wail from here.

Her father wouldn't look at her; he just carried on knocking.

Through the frosted glass, Aida thought she saw a dark shape.

Eventually the door opened and she was looking at David, who looked ill – like he was about to vomit.

The Norwegian doctor had left the spotlight on above the desk in the bedroom and David had woken up suddenly to find himself staring straight into it. Now, wherever he looked, there was a black sun.

Aida saw the man stare at her father then at her. She looked away, down at the ground, smelling the alcohol on him.

'This isn't the one,' her father mumbled, pushing her in front of him as he shuffled across the threshold.

The house was unfinished. Electrical wires stuck out of the wall in clusters, and by the front door a picture of a dolphin hung on bare cement. It was the first time she'd been inside a house for months.

She tried to step back through the front door, but her father had hold of her arm.

'I said I'd come here to see Guy about the visas.'

'Ask this man.'

'I don't know this man – it isn't what we agreed.' She felt her father's grip tightening on her arm.

'All these people are strangers to us. You can get money from this man – you know how to get money from this man,' he insisted.

Then suddenly, without warning, he started to cry.

The old man's tears made the other man scared.

Aida saw him trying to work them out. He thought – because of the bandage on her arm – they'd come looking for a doctor.

'What is it? Are you hurt? Is the girl hurt? OK, OK,' he started saying rapidly, over and over again, but the old man wouldn't shut up. 'OK.'

A door to one side of the hallway was flung open and a man over six feet tall stood there rubbing his eyes.

He yawned and tried to shake himself awake.

Aida heard the man in front of them ask the tall man if he was a doctor.

'Yeah, I'm a doctor, a bloody tired doctor,' Marcus yelled.

Her father, shocked, stopped crying.

'I woke up and heard knocking at the door.'

'I'm surprised you woke up at all. You should have seen the state you were in a few hours ago. You didn't know your own name.'

'Who are you?'

'An MSF doctor – I brought you here from Petri's.'

Aida tried to follow this exchange between the two men – afraid now, and wondering where Guy was.

'Are they from the village?'

The doctor looked at the other man, exhausted. 'They're from the camp. The old man probably paid to get past the perimeter fence and now he's offering us his daughter.'

'He looks pretty upset,' David said. 'And the girl's got some sort of bandage round her arm.'

The doctor yawned again.

'Crocodile tears,' he said then suddenly leant forward and pulled the bandage from Aida's arm, briefly sniffing it. 'What's this?' he asked her in Albanian. 'Pig's blood?'

'Cow,' she mumbled.

Her father persisted in his crying only now, she realised, they were real tears; the frustrated sort he used to cry with her mother when for days on end she refused to speak to him.

The grip on her arm loosened, but she didn't move from the spot.

'Take her, for Jesus' sake,' the doctor suddenly shouted at the other man, pointing to Aida. 'I need sleep.'

Then he disappeared back into his bedroom, slamming the door shut behind him.

After a while her father shuffled backwards through the open front door, leaving her and the man who smelt bad standing on their own in the hallway.

The man took a quick look at her, pushed the door opposite the doctor's room open, and gestured to her to follow.

They were standing in a kitchen.

He found a light above the cooker, switched it on, and took another look at her.

'What's your name?'

She stared at him, but didn't answer.

She'd seen men drunk before – the way they tried to find their way back into themselves – and watched the man in front of her trying to do this now.

'I'm David,' he said.

She hesitated then nodded.

He turned his back on her and started searching the cupboards until he found two cups and a box of sugar cubes.

'I think I'm making coffee – do you want some?' He held up a red enamel jug.

She stepped forwards and pulled the jug out of his hand,

then moved past him towards the hob, and started making the coffee herself.

'Was that your father?' he said, watching her pour the coffee into the cups.

She nodded again.

The hot coffee made him gag and he needed to lie down.

The girl was looking round her like she was waiting for somebody.

In the end, unable to prop himself against the kitchen units any longer, he led the way upstairs back to the room he guessed the doctor must have somehow got him to the night before.

He watched as the girl's gaze shifted nervously about. Not with curiosity, but like a detective in a film, looking for clues in a room where a crime had been committed.

Their eyes lit on Guy's rucksack, propped against the desk legs, at the same time. She watched the man walk hesitantly over, pick it up, open it then put the bag back down on the floor again.

'You were at the party?' she asked, not taking her eyes off him.

'No, I didn't go to the party.'

She wondered if that was where Guy was; if this man knew Guy. She could tell from the way he was looking around him that he was as much of a stranger to the house as she was.

Then she opened her mouth and, looking at the rucksack by the desk, said, 'Guy lives here?'

'Guy? You know Guy?'

He sat down on the bed wanting badly to lie down, but somehow managed to stay sitting.

Hesitantly, she took her headscarf off.

David saw that her hair was short, and the shortness of it felt suddenly wilful – like a trick she had kept hidden up her sleeve.

He looked at her closely for the first time. She had more make-up on than he had realised and was wearing a necklace of what looked like real gold.

She looked nervous, but not afraid.

Then he saw the fear come creeping over her as she watched him thinking; his face changing with his thoughts.

He was sobering up.

'What's your name?' he said again.

Again, she didn't answer him.

He thought about Guy talking to him about the girl – this girl.

He couldn't remember what Guy had said or what he had said, but remembered them talking.

Her father had come to do business with her at night rather than stand by and watch her fall in love in broad daylight. Was she in love? He didn't know, but what he became aware of was an overwhelming sense of destruction rising up inside him.

'You came here looking for Guy?'

She gave a brief nod.

He got up from the bed and went and stood in front of her, as close as if they had been on the underground in rush hour.

She flinched and stepped back, David taking a step forward to every step back she took. Until they hit the wall.

Her back was up against it. He saw her eyes still shifting, assessing the situation. Trying to find not so much a way out as a way through it.

With one hand he started to unbutton her cardigan; the left-hand side of his body pressing against her. Underneath the cardigan she was wearing a T-shirt with *dressed to kill* written on it.

He didn't feel gentle right then, but stroked her face gently because he had never stroked a woman's face in any other way before.

She didn't turn her head away; she was staring straight at him.

He stood looking at her for about a second more then grabbed hold of her wrist, dragging her towards the bed.

Now she resisted.

Neither of them had done this before – they were novices and botched it. He hit his leg against a chair, and she tripped up. He soon got hold of her again by her upper arm this time, pressing his thumbs in hard. Breathing heavily, he also got hold of a handful of hair and was yanking at it, watching her head fall sharply to one side.

Then she came slamming against him, pushing them both on to the bed with her on top.

Her eyes registered hatred, matching his.

With a lot of difficulty he turned her over on the single bed, the weight of his whole body pressing down on her, then she went limp. Everything at once – even her eyes.

David remained poised for a second between the need to give vent to violence, to destroy, and the need to escape.

He was suddenly able to smell himself – too much. He stank of the booze and smoke he had soaked up.

The next second he rolled off her, willing her to come back to life, but she didn't, she just lay there staring up at the ceiling, every now and then her eyelids flickering.

He stood right back from the bed in the middle of the room, but she didn't move.

Then, a second later, her body curled over onto its side and he went running and slipping down the stairs, out into the dawn where there wasn't a living soul to be seen.

In the lobby of Sophia's apartment block, on the wall by the foot of the stairs, there was some new graffiti written in English: Nazi killers go home ⚡. He brushed his hand lightly over it and started to climb the stairs.

Sophia was sitting watching TV in an old dressing gown, her hair in curlers, the sound off. The ash-tray beside her was full.

'You waited up for me?' he whispered.

'I couldn't sleep.'

He sat down next to her, but she didn't take her eyes off the screen, whose flickering light was the only thing moving in the room.

Sophia smelt of cheap bubble bath and cigarettes.

They sat there, not speaking, and after a while she got up and turned off the television.

The room fell into semi-darkness.

He heard her sigh, then say, 'What happened?'

'One day I might tell you.'

Stubbing out her cigarette, she started fishing in the pack open on her lap for another one. 'But not today?'

'Last night I was given a choice – an opportunity to find out more about myself than I ever wanted to know.'

She rattled the empty cigarette box and stood up. 'Night.'

'Sophia.' He caught hold of her hand as she passed. 'Maybe we should get married.'

She gave his hand a quick kiss then left the room.

He waited five minutes more, but she didn't come back so he went into the room he was sleeping in and, lying down on the sofa fully dressed, fell immediately asleep.

He was woken about two hours later by the sound of the lift

mechanism and the springs in the sofa, which began to vibrate as the lift rattled up the shaft.

A shadow crossed the frosted glass and a second later the door to his room slowly opened.

'David?'

He didn't answer.

'You were calling out in your sleep.'

He couldn't remember anything, but his mouth felt dry, as if he had been shouting for a long time.

He heard Sophia's slippers shuffle across the parquet floor as she sat down on the other sofa, beneath her painting of the Last Supper.

He closed his eyes, but could feel her watching him.

She coughed as she slid a book off the coffee table. The dust lay thick and heavy on the cheap furniture in the room.

'*An Atlas of the Crusades* – this kind of thing interests you?' she said in disbelief, flicking through it in the dim light. 'The dream of recovering Jerusalem . . .' she started to read out, then changed her mind and shut the book with a bang.

He opened his eyes.

She said, 'You're awake.'

'The lift woke me.'

'You were having nightmares.'

'I never have nightmares.'

She paused. 'I've heard you most nights since you got here.'

'What are you going to do about it?'

'I thought about recording them so that I'd be able to listen to your voice when you're gone . . . when you're not here any more . . . when you say you'll call, but don't.'

As he sat up, he saw the dim light illuminating the satin of her dressing-gown collar, which was shaped like a scallop shell.

'What about your heart surgeon?'

'David – there is no heart surgeon.'

He waited, knowing enough about her to know that he shouldn't speak at this moment.

'I made him up – that's what you say, isn't it? I like that.' She paused. 'That night you arrived, I went round to a friend's house. I got out of those clothes, washed the make-up off and went to sleep. Somehow managed to get to sleep,' she corrected herself.

After she said this, she looked as though she had shrunk to half her usual size. She shuddered slightly and mumbled something under her breath.

'What do you say in English when that happens? When you shudder suddenly like that?'

'Someone passed over my grave.'

She looked at him, unconvinced.

'I remember, when we first met, you said that you always wondered what the world was going to make of you.'

'I said that?'

'Well, I only ever wondered what I was going to make of the world – I can't help thinking that, without trying, we've somehow ended up at the same point.'

She crossed the immeasurable distance between the two sofas and was kneeling beside him before he knew it, pushing his hair gently from his forehead where it needed cutting. The backdraft from this rapid movement smelt of the perfume he had bought her that day in the mall. She must have been wearing it earlier – had probably been wearing it since the day he bought it for her, only he had never noticed.

'There's something I meant to tell you,' she whispered.

'Save it for later,' he said, his hand touching her face.

'I have to tell you now – if you leave this time, you won't come back.'

'Is that it?'

'No – that's not it. The thing I meant to tell you – whether you stay or go, and just in case I'm not around to tell you when you need to hear it – is that no man dies without consequence. No man.'

30°c and rapidly rising...

12 June 1999 / Russian troops enter Pristina three and a half hours before NATO troops enter Kosovo, and install themselves at the airport — British, French and US K-For troops enter to begin taking control of withdrawing Serb forces

Tomo's mother recognised the girl standing outside in the hallway as soon as she opened the door, and wished she wasn't still wearing her dressing gown.

They stood staring at each other for a moment then Mrs Luković said, 'Come in.'

Violetta walked hesitantly past her, into the apartment and she shut the door, resting briefly against it.

'I'm sorry it's early,' Violetta said.

'It's not early at all — Tomo and his dad sleep in on Saturdays, and I . . .' her voice broke nervously, 'get depressed so I stay in my dressing gown.'

'I do that as well,' Violetta said, smiling. 'When I get depressed.'

'D'you want some coffee?'

'Please.'

A few minutes later Violetta followed her into the kitchen.

Mrs Luković, still nervous, finished clumsily making the coffee while talking to herself under her breath.

Violetta listened to her reassuring herself, 'There now — there we go — right then — here we are', and wanted to lay her hand on the other woman's arm to calm her down, but knew this would only make things worse.

She wished she didn't have this effect on people when she was alone with them — making them nervous.

They took their coffee on to the balcony, which was still in the shade at this time of day.

'Tomo was expecting you?'

'Oh, no – I got some news about the Balkan anthology from the British Council he might want to hear. Good news.'

Mrs Luković only nodded and stared at the apartment blocks opposite.

She took a quick glance at Violetta's long white arms hanging out of the sleeveless black T-shirt and wondered how they stayed so white when the weather was like it was.

A light wind crept round the corner of the building, lifting the hem of Mrs Luković's dressing gown slightly, and making a small football with Goofy on it that used to belong to Tomo roll around in a circle.

Violetta lifted her face to the breeze.

'You seem happy,' Mrs Luković said.

'I am,' Violetta said, turning to her.

She liked the girl's straightforwardness; liked her for not apologising for her happiness.

'Boris told me about you.'

'He did?'

'In the beginning, I mean, when he first found you.'

Tomo's mother sipped at her coffee, smacking her lips slightly. She was getting old.

The sun slanted across the right-hand corner of the balcony, making the solid cement prickle with light.

'I thought he was going to fall in love with you.'

'Maybe he did. Just for a little bit.'

'Just for a little bit,' Mrs Luković agreed, smiling.

'Boris has a great capacity for love,' Violetta said.

'Too great,' Mrs Luković said, with genuine sadness.

Violetta swallowed a mouthful of coffee. She could hear the birds now, as well as dogs barking and the metallic creak of gates; the scuffle of footsteps on the dusty road and cars starting smoothly or with a judder. The sun fell in a solid block across almost half the balcony and she moved her foot into it.

'Boris told me about Berlin,' Mrs Luković said. 'Would you ever go back?'

'To Berlin? No.'

'Never?' Mrs Luković persisted.

'I wouldn't have a reason to.'

'I'd like to go to Berlin.'

Violetta didn't have anything to say to this and for a while they sat in silence.

'I remember one night . . .'

'In Berlin?' Mrs Luković cut in.

Violetta nodded.

'I found this open-air swimming pool. There was an attendant in the kiosk still, but she told me the pool was closed. I couldn't take my eyes off the water – the way it looked under moonlight. So I took a 50DM note out of my purse and held it up against the kiosk window, grinning, waiting. But the woman inside just shook her head. I couldn't believe it – there was the 50DM note pressed against the glass and all she had to do was turn a blind eye while I jumped in the pool and swam around for five minutes or so, but she was shaking her head. She wouldn't take the bribe.'

Violetta stopped talking.

The pegs on the washing line jutting out from the balcony railings shook in the light wind. The same wind blew cigarette smoke up from an apartment below.

The sunlight had already lost its early morning freshness. It had become harsher and more indiscriminate, starting to flatten things – animate and inanimate – into the ground.

The two women sat, contented, noticing all this.

'You know what really got me? What really got me was the reason she refused the bribe. I mean, she didn't refuse it on moral grounds – she refused it because it wasn't in her job description to accept it. It was therefore logical for her to refuse it, and ever since then – that moment standing outside the kiosk with the 50DM note pressed against the window – logic has seemed to me to be predictable, indiscriminate and without morality. Suddenly, I didn't know what I was doing. My world fell apart – it quite literally fell apart.' She paused. 'I'd never felt so homesick.'

Mrs Luković took another sip of coffee, not meaning to smack her lips, but doing it before she could stop herself. 'I'm the first person to hear that, aren't I?' she said.

Violetta nodded.

'D'you feel better now?' she asked. Then, without waiting for a

reply, said, 'You will feel better now you've got it off your chest.'
She smacked her lips again.

The hairdresser on the other side of the street slid back the glass
panels at the front of the salon and a burst of women's voices and
hairdryers filled the air.

'Don't your feet get hot in those boots in the summer?'

Violetta looked down at her black lace-up boots and shrugged.

'You should be wearing sandals.'

'I haven't worn sandals since I was about five.'

'We'll get you some sandals,' Mrs Luković asserted, suddenly
very sure of herself.

The next minute Tomo appeared in his underwear still half-
asleep.

He stared at Violetta and his mother sitting together on the
white plastic garden chairs.

'You OK?' he said, slow with sleep and not knowing what else
to say.

'We're fine,' his mother said. 'Just sitting here putting the world
to rights.'

'Not much then,' he said, yawning.

'Not much,' his mother agreed.

Violetta smiled.

Enver's wife paused in front of the TV, watching it in the way she
always did – like she was looking through it and not at it.

From where Enver was sitting, the plate of salted beef and rice
she was holding protruded across the screen, cutting the image of
crowds at the border in half.

'God knows what they're going back to,' she said.

'Maybe He does, maybe He doesn't,' Enver said impatiently.
'I'm hungry.'

She stared at the screen a moment longer then put the plate
down on the table.

He sat back in the chair, pressing his tie with one hand against
his belly as she moved the dishcloth backwards and forwards over
the table, wiping it. Then she pushed the plate in front of him.

Enver started to eat.

His wife sat at the opposite end of the table and lit a cigarette.
She had dyed her hair the night before – not out of vanity, just for
a change, she said – without reading the instructions properly, and

the bright orange curls had been irritating him all morning. He heard her slip her shoes off and sigh. This was followed by the uneven rustling sound of her rubbing her stockinged feet together.

On the screen they kept getting different bird's-eye views of the queue stretching from the border back to the tolls on the Stengova bypass. The mass of people was unmoving as the collective will of an entire nation was brought to a halt trying to force itself through a bottleneck of less than fifty metres of land.

'It's taking them over four hours to cross through,' she said, tutting and shaking her head. 'They say they're taking their tents down, packing them and walking out of the camps.' She squinted at him through the smoke from her cigarette, appealing to him for confirmation of what was happening in the outside world.

He nodded but didn't say anything.

'In your native land the mud is sweeter than honey,' she said, speaking to herself.

Enver's fork remained poised near his open mouth as he stared at her. She did this every now and again. Showed him glimpses of a more lucid and articulate version of herself that had the ability to reason with chaos. At moments like this, she frightened him and he couldn't help thinking that if she had frightened him more often there might have been more love between them.

He stared at the screen, expecting to see the hordes at the border in a different light, but he couldn't.

'The beef's tough,' he said, trying to chew.

She turned blankly to him, briefly watching his mouth. 'You shouldn't have asked for the salted then – at this time of year you don't have to eat salted. That's last year's anyway.'

He swallowed that mouthful and put another one in.

'There's only so much you can expect from last year's beef.'

He stopped chewing for a moment and stared at her profile. Her sagging chin and pockmarked face with its scattering of warts.

When he was younger he used to joke with his lovers about the number of warts his wife had. But now, two sons and a daughter later, he no longer joked about her warts.

These days, she resolved most village disputes before they even reached his ears and lately Emshi had been happy to leave messages with her without needing to follow them up with him personally.

'Lirije's in love,' she said, still in profile, staring through the motionless masses on the screen at something beyond.

He opened his mouth wider to grind down the last piece of beef. When he'd swallowed it, he sighed.

Sunlight cut in through the window across the TV and in a solid line across the table so that they couldn't look at each other without squinting. He put his hand across his brow to shield his eyes.

'With Spatim,' she said, finishing her sentence.

He brought his hand away from his face and started digging his fork into the pile of rice on his plate.

He pushed forkful after forkful into his mouth, feeling the grease over his lips and trying to work out whether he disliked the idea of Spatim as a son-in-law or not. Then, whether he was supposed to dislike the idea or not. Spatim's father was convicted of second-degree murder and they weren't a good family. He looked at his wife, waiting for a word or look from her that would guide his thoughts.

'You're sure?' he said when nothing was forthcoming.

She seemed frozen to the spot.

He shovelled another forkful of rice in while keeping his eyes on her and watching for any sign of movement.

'You should talk to her,' she said at last.

The sunlight had shifted round so that it was now falling over the empty plate, his right elbow and upper arm. In the silence that followed his wife's pronouncement it reached his right shoulder.

The half of him not in sunlight felt cold.

'You don't know her.'

'I don't, do I?' Enver agreed. Then, after a while, added, 'I'm sorry.'

'But you do know love.'

He stared at her, becoming more frightened by the second, then looked down at the few remaining grains of rice lying in the grease on his plate, because they looked familiar and reassuring.

'I know both of you – I know she loves like you love – like you're in love, now.' She sounded almost contented. 'She knows how to risk everything – I don't know how to do that.'

With a clatter that shook Enver completely, she picked up his plate and plodded with her heavy ankles and heavy body back towards the kitchen.

The sunlight fell directly over him, illuminating and temporarily blinding him.

'You should talk to her,' she said again from behind the kitchen door.

The 4x4 ground to a halt, temporarily forming the tail-end of a queue of traffic stretching from the tolls to the border.

'It could be three hours from here.'

Howard switched the engine off and turned to look at Donatella, who had her bare feet up on the dashboard so that she could apply aloe vera gel to her sunburnt legs.

She looked briefly out of the window, wincing, then back down at her legs.

He stared out at the billboards in front of the petrol station on the opposite side of the road. A half-naked woman on a mobile phone advertising Mobimak telecommunications; a man in a suit looking for a cure for something in a Zegin pharmacy. And a new poster he hadn't seen before for Republika Foods, showing the footbridge over the Vardar and a man standing up on the parapet about to commit suicide. The slogan read: Life is Beautiful. He smiled and pointed it out to Donatella.

'Someone with a sense of humour,' she said, keeping her legs stretched out because it hurt too much to bend them. 'Hope I can still walk.'

'I'll carry you if you can't.'

'You're just saying that,' she said, knowing he meant it.

Twenty minutes later, he switched the engine back on and they crawled along, kilometre after kilometre, in second gear. Donatella stared out of the open window at the people on the road, for faces she might recognise from Stengova camp. Neither she nor Howard thought of offering a lift to anyone – of filling up the empty seats in the back of the jeep.

'Chris tried to get them to take the tents down so that we could clean and pack them and send them into Kosovo in one consignment, but they're just walking out with them. If they'd only waited until official UNHCR repatriation on 1st July, this mess could have been avoided.'

'Who's going to stand up and tell them that? I think they're outside the realm of memos and brainstorming sessions. You remember Arsim in the camp? He crossed over the border a week ago then came back to Stengova to tell his wife their house was burnt to the ground. Within an hour she'd packed up everything they had – ready to go – house or no house. You can't stop this now.' He looked out of the window.

They reached the border at midday and made their way to the aid post Women Against War was sharing with World Refugee Council.

Howard went straight over to the temporary toilet blocks, which were overflowing.

The fresh food distribution point had been overrun within the first hour of operation and they'd virtually run out of family food packs. Genevieve was trying to appease people by handing out baby kits from surplus stock, but wasn't feeling well and every now and then had to keep disappearing in order to be sick.

The tent Donatella was meant to be giving mine-awareness talks in was full of women and children forced to convert it into overflow toilet facilities when the blocks were closed down.

Donatella stepped back out into the sun. The skin on her legs was so tight it felt as if it was shrinking and there wasn't enough to cover the bone, muscle and tissue. They were prickling and she had to resist the urge to scratch. She needed to get out of the sun, but there was no shade.

Six MI-24 helicopters flew overhead.

She watched staff from the prevention of parent-child separation team moving among the crowd in their bright white T-shirts and sunglasses, vital and ineffectual.

Nadia passed briefly across her field of vision, pursuing a young woman with a child clamped to her hip. Unexpected budget surplus meant that she was given the go-ahead for psycho-social counselling at the border.

'What's wrong with Genevieve?' Donatella called out.

'Morning sickness,' Nadia shouted back.

The MI-24s flew back the other way.

The air was charged with an anticipation that was trying to outbalance a fatal sense of loss.

The mass of people who had, months before, clung to life on the same patch of land, now crackled with it. She knew this scene, which was part of a cyclical process and never changed.

She stood looking out over them at the brown and grey humps of mountain, noticing the mountains now for the first time because she wanted to be on the other side of them.

Then she shifted her gaze to the toilet blocks where she'd last seen Howard. There he was with some kind of wrench in his hand and a team of reluctant volunteers. No longer interested, she turned back to face the mountains.

She'd be back in a week's time, with her passport, ready to cross the border.

Guy drove past the new supermarket and its garden furniture display, into the motel forecourt.

The heat was unbearable once the car stopped. His clothes stuck to him and the air smelt of oil. The afternoon felt inflammable and he wouldn't have been surprised to see – reflected in Aida's sunglasses – the motel behind them going up in flames.

He took her hand and helped her out of the car, her breasts brushing against his arm as she moved past him. She was wearing a lot of make-up that showed no sign of melting in the heat.

They crossed the shifting forecourt and strip of unfinished pavement running along the front of the motel then climbed the white marble steps up to reception.

The mirror glass made the world outside look grey; as though a storm was continually brewing. It didn't look like the world they had just come from.

They waited for a while by the reception desk, but nobody came. A fax machine started bleeping and Guy watched as several sheets of paper slipped through and fell over the side of the desk on to the floor. He read the framed sign up on the wall, written in English, German, Macedonian and Albanian. All rooms came with French beds. There was a nightly rate and an hourly rate. He tried to remember if he had ever stayed in a hotel where hourly rates were charged.

'D'you want something to drink?' he said at last.

Aida nodded and followed him across the white tiled floor into the bar.

The back wall hadn't been completed and there was plastic sheeting stretched across the hole. Taxes weren't paid on incomplete buildings.

The bar was full.

Guy recognised several internationals from the camp, but nobody he knew by name.

A waiter brought them a beer and a Coca-Cola.

Through the glass-top table, Guy watched Aida cross and uncross her legs.

There was a piano playing somewhere, but he couldn't work out whether it was live or recorded. He couldn't decide whether the plants were fake or real either.

He turned to Aida, but she was looking around her, more interested in what the girls in the bar were wearing than anything else. He had never known anyone ask so few questions before or go to such lengths to safeguard their curiosity. She had got into the car at noon without once asking where they were going and had got out of it just now in the motel forecourt and walked into reception without a single comment.

The piano stopped playing and was replaced by dimly recognisable rock music.

'Were you here before?' she said suddenly.

Her quickening grasp of English terrified him because it was connected to her will, which was beyond his comprehension and vice-like.

'Never.' He ordered himself another beer.

She turned away, nonplussed by his reassurance, but her hand shook every time it reached out for the glass of Coca-Cola.

'Have you?' he said after a while.

She stared back at him, thinking, and didn't reply.

He had to stop himself from asking again.

He finished his beer and stood up. She finished the last of her Coca-Cola.

They slid back over the white tiles into reception.

There was a man standing behind the desk now. In a waistcoat made out of the same fabric that the chairs were covered in.

'I'd like a room please,' Guy said, his voice breaking, feeling childish. 'You do have rooms – vacancies, I mean?'

'Of course.' The receptionist nodded slowly, looking past him at Aida. 'You want standard or executive?'

Guy hesitated, feeling cornered. 'Executive.'

'Of course,' the man said again. 'With French bed?'

Guy looked at the sign on the wall again. 'Don't they all come with French beds?'

'Of course,' the receptionist said, waiting.

'Well . . .'

'So you want executive room with French bed – you have passport?'

'No.' Guy stared blankly at him. He had completely forgotten about his passport.

The receptionist thought about this – aware he held the other man's world in his hands – making him wait.

'Credit cards?'

'Yes, I have credit cards,' Guy said, excited, passing three over the counter.

The receptionist inspected all of them, keeping the American Express and handing the others back.

'One night?'

'One night.'

He put the credit card down carefully next to the telephone then turned round and hooked a key off the wall.

'So – I show you.'

They followed him across reception and up several flights of stairs. From the outside the motel hadn't looked high enough to conceal so many twists in the staircase. He heard Aida's steady tread on the thin carpet behind him.

The receptionist put the key in a door with the number 142 on it.

They walked into a small hallway with a minuscule bathroom leading off it.

'If you want a shower you must use this switch to heat water. The water it takes one – maybe two hours to heat. So,' he said, flicking the switch up. The red light on the boiler lit up orange.

Then he opened a second door leading into the bedroom.

The bed occupied almost the entire room, and there was just enough space between the foot of the bed and the wall to walk round from one side to the other.

The window was ceiling to floor and covered in an expanse of netting.

'This is the executive room?' Guy asked.

'Of course,' the receptionist said, pointing to the mirror on the wall at the foot of the bed. 'You like the room? You happy?'

'Happier than I've ever been in my life before,' Guy said, straight-faced.

The receptionist paused then left, putting the key in the door, which he left open.

A woman with bleached blonde hair wearing rubber clogs pushed a vacuum cleaner slowly up the hallway outside, then Guy shut the door.

The room had no air conditioning and he tried to find a way behind the net curtains to see if he could open the window, but soon gave up.

Aida stood on the other side of the bed, watching him.

'We stay here?'

'If you like,' he said, turning to face her, his knees knocking against the bed frame.

'I like.'

'Good.'

'We stay here tonight also?'

'Maybe.'

She thought about this, her arms hanging down by her sides.

'We go back to the camp?'

'Maybe.'

'Maybe not?'

He shrugged. 'Maybe not.'

'I have no clothes – nothing.'

He watched her for a second longer then squeezed past the end of the bed, his shoulder sending the executive mirror swinging on the wall, and went into the bathroom, shutting the door and locking it then sat down on the closed toilet lid, taking in the wall-to-wall peach tiling and breathing deeply.

The soap in the dish was packaged in shiny white paper with a crown painted on it. He took hold of it, turning it over in his hands.

The bathroom reminded him of the loos at the Italian restaurant he used to go to in Guildford. He remembered going there one Friday night, after a week when he had managed to sell four flats on a strip of road that was about to cave in because of an ancient chalk pit. Shortly after the road did cave in, a young couple he sold one of the flats to were evacuated and – he later found out – the husband committed suicide in their emergency accommodation: a badly run bed and breakfast. He tried to get in contact with the girl afterwards, but she refused to see him.

He got up from the toilet seat, unlocked the bathroom door and went back into the bedroom.

Aida was standing by the curtains watching the traffic on the road outside.

The room was full of her silence.

He sat down on the bed. It creaked and felt as though it would break in half.

She turned round to watch him.

He picked the phone up from the bedside table and dialled reception, watching her back.

'You do room service?'

'Of course,' the receptionist's now familiar voice said.

'I want champagne.'

'Of course – French or Croatian?'

Guy laughed.

The receptionist didn't.

'Make it French.'

He was still sitting on the bed and Aida was still standing by the window when the receptionist knocked and came into the room with the champagne.

He walked over to the widescreen TV and put the tray on top of it.

'You want I pour it?'

Guy nodded and watched as the man popped the cork and poured the champagne.

As the cork popped, Aida jumped, laughing at herself.

It was the first time he had ever heard her laugh.

Still laughing, she said something to the receptionist, who smiled.

He left the two glasses of champagne on the tray and the bottle in the bucket.

Guy got up from the bed to tip him and saw from the man's sneer that he had tipped too much. Tipping too much had the same effect here as not tipping at all. In fact it was probably better not to tip at all.

'What did you say to him?' he asked Aida when the receptionist had left.

She repeated what she had said.

'In English,' Guy said.

'In English I don't know how to say.'

He thought about the day at Mavro and how much she had changed since then. In Mavro she had been making her mind up – now she had made it up. He didn't want to know how.

He picked the two glasses up from the tray. 'I want you to drink this.'

She nodded and took the glass held out to her.

He realised, watching her take her first sip, that he could take her away with him and she would come. She would never relinquish her will to survive and he would never relinquish his love for her. This is what would make their lives.

She would be the one thing he suffered, relentlessly. Every meal no matter how sumptuous, every bouquet no matter how exotic, and every present no matter how bejewelled, would all mean nothing to her. She would never love him, and yet she would never be able to outlive his love for her either.

He sat next to her on the bed.

'You're coming with me,' he said.

She nodded.

They sat, carefully watching each other, drinking the champagne.

Flora stood at the kitchen window, which overlooked a garden her reduced rent didn't grant her access to. It looked full and busy with life – like it had its own agenda. The owner of the small apartment block, a woman with brown hair the same colour as her dachshund, appeared with a basket of washing and began to peg a sheet on the line, the dog yapping round her ankles, squeaking every now and then as she trod on it.

Feeling vaguely resentful, Flora moved away from the window and made herself a coffee.

She went through to the lounge, careful to put the TV guide under her cup. She'd once left a cup on the coffee table and gone out. When she arrived back at the apartment, the cup was gone and on the table instead was a note from the landlady saying that she wasn't to put things directly on to surfaces because it ruined the varnish. The woman had been into her flat during the day without her permission. Had watched through the grille in the basement wall where she lived, at the bottom of the building, for Flora's feet to appear; watched them walk along the cement path leading to the front gate; listened to the gate squeaking on its hinges then gone up the stairs, let herself in and had a good poke around. Flora could see her doing this, clearly.

She paid her money every month on time and it brought her neither privacy nor freedom – so what was the point? She thought about getting the locks changed on her front door; she thought about going down to the woman's basement apartment and giving vent to her anger.

The woman had been back since. Had moved things every time – just small objects – so that Flora would know she'd been, and after every intrusion she felt outrage, but did nothing.

She switched the TV on in time to see clips from yesterday's episode of *Sunset Boulevard*, bringing viewers who had missed that instalment up to date – this took about eight seconds. The familiar music burst out of the screen and Flora sat on the edge of the sofa with anticipation, hunched over her coffee and cigarette.

She was in love with Roberto, who had found out – only yesterday – that he had a ten-year-old son he never knew about. She found herself humming along to the theme tune, which was fading out, when the telephone started to ring.

She felt justified in not answering it. This was her one hour of reprieve during the day, spent in the hot-blooded jumble of lives on Buenos Aires's Sunset Boulevard, and she remained sitting on the edge of the sofa.

Roberto walked up and down the street in front of the house he now knew his son lived in. His wife passed in her car, pulled up on the opposite kerb and called out to him. At that moment some curtains at one of the windows in the house were pulled back.

The phone stopped ringing.

Roberto's wife looked at him, then past his shoulder at the house behind him. There was a woman at the window, a beautiful woman. Roberto's wife looked first at him then at the beautiful woman in the house behind.

Her face changed.

It changed again when the front door opened and a young boy stepped out on to the porch.

Roberto spun round on his heels.

Flora muttered to herself.

The phone started ringing again. It sounded more urgent this time even though she knew phones couldn't do that.

The beautiful woman disappeared from the window and re-appeared a second later in the doorway behind the boy, her hands on his shoulders. They both stood there staring at Roberto and his wife, and Roberto and his wife stared back. A stand-off.

A sprinkler started up on the front lawn. Flora noticed that the rolled-up sleeves of Roberto's shirt got wet. He must have been standing too near the sprinkler – she didn't like to think of him being careless.

She pushed herself up from the sofa and walked over to where the phone hung on the wall, still ringing.

Her eyes never once leaving the screen, she picked up the receiver.

'Hello?'

Through the crackle, she made out another 'hello'. It sounded like an echo of her own that had got lost.

'Hello?' she said again, slowly turning away from the screen. Less impatient now.

'Flora?'

Her name got broken up and it took a while for all the pieces to make their way down the line.

'Hello?' she said again, even though she'd recognised the man's voice.

'Flora,' he said.

This time it wasn't the line breaking up.

She waited, still needing to hear her name a third time.

'Flora?'

'Dad?'

It felt more like she'd swallowed the word than spoken it. She wondered who had decreed, in the beginning, that nouns – above any other words – should have the power to conceal the unique within the universal.

'Where are you?'

'Priština – I'm using a Russian officer's phone.'

He paused.

She listened.

'We're alive,' he managed to say at last.

It was everything, but it wasn't enough. She stared down at her feet in their socks.

'I have to go – we'll call you again later.'

Nothing else.

The line went down, but she stayed standing near the phone, her shoulder against the wall, the receiver still pressed against her ear. A recorded voice told her to hang up and try again.

She did as the voice said, hung up and moved slowly over to the sofa, sitting back down again.

Her coffee was cold.

She leant forwards and picked up a handful of peanuts from the dish on the table.

Roberto was sitting in his Ferrari, parked outside his son's school, looking more like a stalker than a long-lost father.

Flora sat on the edge of the sofa, her hand going to her mouth, her mouth chewing the peanuts until she wasn't able to chew any more because she had started to cry and the hand holding the peanuts was shaking uncontrollably.

Harvey was still suffering from the shock of finding Val in reception that afternoon. Standing with her elbows on the desk in white and beige weekend casual with a red suitcase beside her.

He approached her with caution, unsure whether she would explode on contact.

'This woman – she is your wife?' the receptionist said – the one Harvey had been wanting to thump in the face for as long as he could remember.

He stared at Val and didn't answer.

She'd changed her hair, and her eyes looked different. She looked somehow smarter – sharper.

'She is your wife?' the receptionist repeated.

'I guess,' Harvey said, turning quickly to Val as he realised what he had just said.

But she was laughing – really laughing – like he was really funny. 'Oh, Harvey,' she said.

He let the breath whistle out of him and asked if she wanted to take the suitcase up to the room. She said, no, she wanted a drink and followed him into the Emperor's Bar, trundling the suitcase after her.

They sat at the fringes of the half-full bar; at a table near the window overlooking the wasteland at the back of the hotel, where there was a line of large metal wheelie bins and, in the distance, the new all-weather tennis court.

'At the airport this hotel – the Aleksandar Palace – was advertised as a hotel for sportsmen – is that a sign of prestige or something?'

'Not that I'm aware of. They probably meant something entirely different and just translated it wrong.'

She asked him to order, which he did, then sat back in her chair.

He was fiddling with everything on the table – sugar cubes, ash-trays, drink mats.

'You crossed the Atlantic,' he said at last.

'It's kind of a necessary part of the journey.'

'I mean – it's the first time you ever crossed it.'

'Yeah, it's something isn't it?'

'How did you do it?' Harvey asked.

'I got on a plane.'

That wasn't what he meant, but she knew that.

They smiled at each other and it suddenly occurred to him, looking at her, that she'd come to tell him something. That she'd crossed the Atlantic so that she could have the satisfaction of telling him – face to face – she was filing for divorce. He kept expecting – every time she shifted in her chair – for her to dig into the pockets of her beige pants and draw out a piece of paper headed Goldburn, Fowler and Vanderholt, and for her to read out in her rasping voice Mr Fowler's apocalyptic correspondence. But no piece of paper emerged and anyway, Val didn't seem to talk like that any more – or maybe she did and it just didn't bother him so much.

The waiter fastidiously wiped the table and arranged the drink mats with one hand. The other hand balanced the tray with the two rakis on it.

The rakis were at long last set down.

'He's had professional training,' Val said, watching the man with open admiration. 'I like to see that.'

She seemed to enjoy the raki more because of it.

'So this is what they drink here?'

'Mostly,' he said, resisting the urge to down it in one go, then not resisting. This curiosity was – like the hair and the eyes – a new thing.

She watched him then did the same.

'More?' he asked, encouraged.

She nodded, wiping her mouth with the back of her hand.

They watched through the window as a Roma woman pushed an empty pram up to the row of bins. Three children under the age of eight trundled after her, the youngest diving into the first bin. Three minutes later his head popped up again out of the top of the rubbish, grinning. His mother turned round and grinned back then started to sift through the overflow pile building up around the bottom of the bins with the two older children.

'Does Lou hate me?' he said at last.

'Lou? No – she disapproves of you.'

'Disapproves?' Harvey said, trying to work this one out.

'I never knew, but in tenth grade apparently they were encouraged to find themselves an ex-Communist pen-pal and Lou wound up with a girl from Belgrade. Can you believe that? I don't think I've ever stuck an airmail sticker on an envelope before and there's my little girl writing to Belgrade. She's gotten very anti-NATO, Harvey,' she explained gently, as if he might not understand.

He sat there nodding and waiting for her to get to the point.

'Your transmissions were pretty pro-war.'

'They were?'

'You really went for it, Harvey.'

'I did? So you watched them?'

'Sure – all of them.' She paused. 'Can you get anything other than salted peanuts?'

He called the waiter over and somehow managed to cajole a dish of fried mushrooms and a basket of bread out of him.

'Lou thinks she's right – on the side of the righteous – and you're wrong. She's been getting it straight from Belgrade.'

'She's growing up,' Harvey said smiling, interested in the fact for the first time.

'She is grown-up – she's eighteen.'

'I'm not letting her go just yet.'

The sun moved round.

'You know what she said to me the other day driving to the airport?'

'Lou drove you to the airport?'

Val nodded. 'She said that the thing about the truth is, the more you're told, the more you're aware of what you're not being told.'

'Lou said that?'

At some point they changed from raki to champagne because it felt right.

Light-headed from jet lag and a diet that consisted so far that day of nothing but bar snacks, Val leant forwards and said, 'Why did you marry me, Harvey?' When he didn't answer, she added, 'It's not a trick question.'

'You smelt different to all the girls I knew. Even the virgins where I grew up smelt stale.'

A flicker of a smile.

'Want to know why I said yes?'

'Don't tell me I smelt stale.'

'You did smell stale – I'd never smelt that on a man before.'

She took his hand to reassure him.

'I never thought you'd say yes,' he said. 'I still can't quite believe you did. I can't believe you're here – now.'

Outside the window the quality of the light changed.

They drank more champagne.

Harvey stared across at Val; Lake Drive Val in her weekend casual but with different hair and different eyes, who had got on a plane and crossed the Atlantic then Europe in order to come looking for him in the lobby of the Aleksander Palace Hotel.

It was like he was about to start having an affair with his wife.

'Your mother's coming?' David asked as he watched the old woman shuffle out of the apartment after them.

'She says she wants to see an old friend.'

'On top of the mountain?'

'The monastery, David.'

'The monastery's now a restaurant serving bad food in historic surroundings – are you going to tell her or am I?'

'The monks relocated about a quarter of a kilometre along the shoulder of the mountain.'

'Your mother's friends with monks?'

'A monk.'

He sighed and they waited for the lift.

'She wants people in the street to see her getting into the new red Fiat,' Sophia said.

They got to the car – Sophia's mother walking so slowly the whole thing began to feel processional. It took both David and Sophia to feed her and her walking stick into the back seat where she spread herself out, commandeering all of it.

'I hate the smell of new cars,' she said as they drove through the town past the General Hospital and half-way up the mountain.

'Has she ever been in one before?' David asked.

'Course not,' Sophia said.

He caught her mother's eye in the rear-view mirror and they smiled at each other. It was like he'd caught sight of a part of Sophia in her and he felt himself warming to the old woman for the first time.

The car park – usually full on a Sunday – was virtually empty apart from a few cars belonging to walkers, and the old man with his red popcorn machine.

David bought a bag for each of them, feeling sorry for the old man standing beside his machine, still full of popcorn at the end of a quiet day.

The shadows were just beginning to lengthen, but there were at least three hours of light left. Enough to get to the top of the mountain and back down again. He had climbed Vodna once before, in winter, when the main aim of the climb was to reach the tea hut at the top, drink cups of clear, sweetened mountain tea, and eat chocolate. The snow had been so thick then that he had slid all the way back down, making it in under an hour.

Leaving Sophia's mother on a bench overlooking the city where she'd agreed to meet her monk, the bag of popcorn on her lap, they started to climb.

The forest was full of the constant sound of crickets, which became maddening if you stood still for too long. They followed the small track as it steadily began to rise, keeping a look out for the deer, boar and other animals that roamed the forest, in order to take their minds off the heat. Within fifteen minutes David's skin was wet and prickling.

They walked through forest for about an hour until the pines gave way to a slope of scrub where bees kept passing low overhead. The path which, in the forest, had been barely a track, broadened into a narrow road full of winter frost craters. The stretch of road lasted for a mile and wound past a house surrounded by barbed wire with a sentry-post at the gates. It looked like the sort of house a once despotic, now retired army general might live in. Somewhere to carry out very private trains of thought, and indulge in very private whims. The house marked the end of the road, which soon became nothing more than a track again, veering away to follow the lower ridge to the summit.

They passed a trio of elderly climbers heading back down and exchanged greetings with them in the good-natured way of people in lonely places.

Then they carried on along the ridge, which was slow work, hand in hand. Nothing but mountains lay in all directions. The valley in which the city lay was hidden from view by the mountain's northern flank. The world felt uncultivated, uncivilised and limitless.

Just ahead the tea hut came into view. It grew up out of the outcrop of rocks on the summit and was circular in shape with radio masts protruding from the roof. On the western side of the outcrop there was a small plateau with a low stone wall round its perimeter, and inside the wall some tables and chairs. To the generous mind, it looked like a garden in a wilderness.

Every now and then David heard snatches of song – an unaccompanied clear voice – but couldn't work out where it was coming from.

'My mother's monk's an old beau,' Sophia said, listening to the voice as well.

'Before your father?'

'Before him – yes.'

'She said "no" and that's why he became a monk?'

'That's what happened,' Sophia said, nodding.

Ten minutes later they reached the tea hut, which was still open.

The main room was large and circular, its grey stone walls unplastered. The stove in the centre was unlit, but the air still smelt faintly of melting snow as it did in winter. They walked over to the kitchen hatch where a cauldron of tea sat steaming, and a man in a cap ladled some of the tea into two plastic cups. On the wall above the hatch there were framed photographs of walkers, and the erection, just behind the tea hut, of a flagpole to fly the then new Republic's flag.

Benches and tables ran like the spokes of a wheel all the way round the room. They chose a bench with a north-west view, but it didn't matter. Mountains lay beyond every window. There was only one other man in the room.

'Can you stay here overnight?'

'Don't even think about it,' Sophia mumbled through a mouthful of chocolate.

He wiped some chocolate saliva from the corner of her mouth and sucked his thumb thoughtfully. Then he took hold of her ear between his thumb and forefinger, and was pulling her towards him when a light suddenly flashed.

He whipped round.

The man who had been sitting down with his back to the room when they arrived was now on his feet with a camera clapped against his face.

'I take picture of you,' he said, letting the camera fall against his chest. Then he smiled, but the smile looked oversized because he was so scrawny. 'You want to buy picture?'

David didn't, but knew – looking at Sophia – that it would mean something if he didn't.

The camera clicked and a Polaroid came out the bottom of it. The man smiled at the picture, making David want to snatch it out of his hand.

'Is good picture.'

Sophia turned round, smiling.

'How much?' David asked.

The man quickly finished his tea with short nervous slurps, the picture on the table beside him, his hand over it.

'Two hundred dinars,' he said.

'Two hundred dinars?'

Sophia looked disappointed in him – there was even a tinge of sadness.

'OK,' he said, trying to sound good-natured.

'You buy?'

'Yes – I buy.'

The man got an envelope out of his bag and pushed the photograph into it. Sealing the envelope, he handed it to David.

Once he had his money he picked up his bag and hurriedly left.

The man in the cap who had served them their tea was watching through the hatch.

David walked back over to the table and opened the envelope.

He pulled out the photograph.

It was blank.

He turned to the man in the hatch, who had known because he'd seen it done before and wanted to see David's face as he opened the envelope.

Then he turned to Sophia, who was laughing.

'Can you believe it?' he said. 'Taking our photograph – asking us to pay for it and nothing – blank.'

'You have to believe it,' Sophia said. 'This is the Balkans.'

They went outside, taking in deep breaths of mountain air. It was much colder and the sun had left the garden. An unspoken mutual idea that they should sit on the summit and watch the sun go down had hung between them all afternoon, but now they were no longer interested in the sunset and started to make their way rapidly back down the mountain, laughing.

From the tea hut on the summit of Vodna, a man and woman could be seen scrambling as fast as they could back down the ridge and upper slopes, breaking into a run as they disappeared into the forest.

Acknowledgements

My thanks – as always – to Rebecca Carter at Chatto for her boundless enthusiasm and commitment, and also to Clare Alexander at Gillon Aitken Associates.

There are so many people without whom this book would not have been possible . . . untold amounts of gratitude go to all the friends we made in Cegrane, Llojane and Skopje who shared their stories and made us feel less like strangers in a foreign land.